ATS-149   ADMISSION TEST SERIES

This is your
PASSBOOK for...

Pharmacy Technician Certification Exam (PTCE)

Test Preparation Study Guide
Questions & Answers

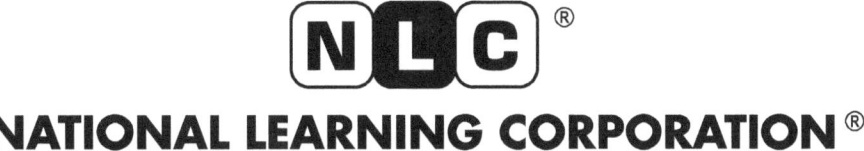

COPYRIGHT NOTICE

This book is SOLELY intended for, is sold ONLY to, and its use is RESTRICTED to individual, bona fide applicants or candidates who qualify by virtue of having seriously filed applications for appropriate license, certificate, professional and/or promotional advancement, higher school matriculation, scholarship, or other legitimate requirements of education and/or governmental authorities.

This book is NOT intended for use, class instruction, tutoring, training, duplication, copying, reprinting, excerption, or adaptation, etc., by:

1) Other publishers
2) Proprietors and/or Instructors of "Coaching" and/or Preparatory Courses
3) Personnel and/or Training Divisions of commercial, industrial, and governmental organizations
4) Schools, colleges, or universities and/or their departments and staffs, including teachers and other personnel
5) Testing Agencies or Bureaus
6) Study groups which seek by the purchase of a single volume to copy and/or duplicate and/or adapt this material for use by the group as a whole without having purchased individual volumes for each of the members of the group
7) Et al.

Such persons would be in violation of appropriate Federal and State statutes.

PROVISION OF LICENSING AGREEMENTS – Recognized educational, commercial, industrial, and governmental institutions and organizations, and others legitimately engaged in educational pursuits, including training, testing, and measurement activities, may address request for a licensing agreement to the copyright owners, who will determine whether, and under what conditions, including fees and charges, the materials in this book may be used them. In other words, a licensing facility exists for the legitimate use of the material in this book on other than an individual basis. However, it is asseverated and affirmed here that the material in this book CANNOT be used without the receipt of the express permission of such a licensing agreement from the Publishers. Inquiries re licensing should be addressed to the company, attention rights and permissions department.

All rights reserved, including the right of reproduction in whole or in part, in any form or by any means, electronic or mechanical, including photocopying, recording, or by any information storage and retrieval system, without permission in writing from the Publisher.

Copyright © 2024 by
National Learning Corporation

212 Michael Drive, Syosset, NY 11791
(516) 921-8888 • www.passbooks.com
E-mail: info@passbooks.com

PASSBOOK® SERIES

THE *PASSBOOK® SERIES* has been created to prepare applicants and candidates for the ultimate academic battlefield – the examination room.

At some time in our lives, each and every one of us may be required to take an examination – for validation, matriculation, admission, qualification, registration, certification, or licensure.

Based on the assumption that every applicant or candidate has met the basic formal educational standards, has taken the required number of courses, and read the necessary texts, the *PASSBOOK® SERIES* furnishes the one special preparation which may assure passing with confidence, instead of failing with insecurity. Examination questions – together with answers – are furnished as the basic vehicle for study so that the mysteries of the examination and its compounding difficulties may be eliminated or diminished by a sure method.

This book is meant to help you pass your examination provided that you qualify and are serious in your objective.

The entire field is reviewed through the huge store of content information which is succinctly presented through a provocative and challenging approach – the question-and-answer method.

A climate of success is established by furnishing the correct answers at the end of each test.

You soon learn to recognize types of questions, forms of questions, and patterns of questioning. You may even begin to anticipate expected outcomes.

You perceive that many questions are repeated or adapted so that you can gain acute insights, which may enable you to score many sure points.

You learn how to confront new questions, or types of questions, and to attack them confidently and work out the correct answers.

You note objectives and emphases, and recognize pitfalls and dangers, so that you may make positive educational adjustments.

Moreover, you are kept fully informed in relation to new concepts, methods, practices, and directions in the field.

You discover that you are actually taking the examination all the time: you are preparing for the examination by "taking" an examination, not by reading extraneous and/or supererogatory textbooks.

In short, this PASSBOOK®, used directedly, should be an important factor in helping you to pass your test.

PHARMACY TECHNICIAN CERTIFICATION EXAM

The Pharmacy Technician Certification Exam (PTCE) is a two-hour, multiple-choice, exam that contains 90 questions (80 scored questions and 10 unscored questions). Each question is shown with four possible answers, only one of which is the correct or best answer. Unscored questions are not identified and are randomly distributed throughout the exam. A candidate's exam score is based on the responses to the 80 scored questions. One hour and 50 minutes are allotted for answering the exam questions and 10 minutes for a tutorial and post-exam survey.

The PTCE assesses knowledge critical to pharmacy technician practice organized into nine knowledge domains, each with a number of 'knowledge areas' or sub-domains, as shown in the table below.

PTCE Blueprint Domains

Knowledge Domains	Domains Description	% of PTCE Content	Knowledge Areas
1	Pharmacology for Technicians	13.75	6
2	Pharmacy Law and Regulations	12.50	15
3	Sterile and Non-Sterile Compounding	8.75	7
4	Medication Safety	12.50	6
5	Pharmacy Quality Assurance	7.50	5
6	Medication Order Entry and Fill Process	17.50	7
7	Pharmacy Inventory Management	8.75	5
8	Pharmacy Billing and Reimbursement	8.75	5
9	Pharmacy Information Systems Usage and Application	10.00	2

For information regarding PTCE contact

Pharmacy Technician Certification Board
2215 Constitution Avenue NW, Suite 101
Washington DC 20037

HOW TO TAKE A TEST

You have studied long, hard and conscientiously.

With your official admission card in hand, and your heart pounding, you have been admitted to the examination room.

You note that there are several hundred other applicants in the examination room waiting to take the same test.

They all appear to be equally well prepared.

You know that nothing but your best effort will suffice. The "moment of truth" is at hand: you now have to demonstrate objectively, in writing, your knowledge of content and your understanding of subject matter.

You are fighting the most important battle of your life—to pass and/or score high on an examination which will determine your career and provide the economic basis for your livelihood.

What extra, special things should you know and should you do in taking the examination?

I. YOU MUST PASS AN EXAMINATION

A. WHAT EVERY CANDIDATE SHOULD KNOW
Examination applicants often ask us for help in preparing for the written test. What can I study in advance? What kinds of questions will be asked? How will the test be given? How will the papers be graded?

B. HOW ARE EXAMS DEVELOPED?
Examinations are carefully written by trained technicians who are specialists in the field known as "psychological measurement," in consultation with recognized authorities in the field of work that the test will cover. These experts recommend the subject matter areas or skills to be tested; only those knowledges or skills important to your success on the job are included. The most reliable books and source materials available are used as references. Together, the experts and technicians judge the difficulty level of the questions.
Test technicians know how to phrase questions so that the problem is clearly stated. Their ethics do not permit "trick" or "catch" questions. Questions may have been tried out on sample groups, or subjected to statistical analysis, to determine their usefulness.
Written tests are often used in combination with performance tests, ratings of training and experience, and oral interviews. All of these measures combine to form the best-known means of finding the right person for the right job.

II. HOW TO PASS THE WRITTEN TEST

A. BASIC STEPS

1) Study the announcement

How, then, can you know what subjects to study? Our best answer is: "Learn as much as possible about the class of positions for which you've applied." The exam will test the knowledge, skills and abilities needed to do the work.

Your most valuable source of information about the position you want is the official exam announcement. This announcement lists the training and experience qualifications. Check these standards and apply only if you come reasonably close to meeting them. Many jurisdictions preview the written test in the exam announcement by including a section called "Knowledge and Abilities Required," "Scope of the Examination," or some similar heading. Here you will find out specifically what fields will be tested.

2) Choose appropriate study materials

If the position for which you are applying is technical or advanced, you will read more advanced, specialized material. If you are already familiar with the basic principles of your field, elementary textbooks would waste your time. Concentrate on advanced textbooks and technical periodicals. Think through the concepts and review difficult problems in your field.

These are all general sources. You can get more ideas on your own initiative, following these leads. For example, training manuals and publications of the government agency which employs workers in your field can be useful, particularly for technical and professional positions. A letter or visit to the government department involved may result in more specific study suggestions, and certainly will provide you with a more definite idea of the exact nature of the position you are seeking.

3) Study this book!

III. KINDS OF TESTS

Tests are used for purposes other than measuring knowledge and ability to perform specified duties. For some positions, it is equally important to test ability to make adjustments to new situations or to profit from training. In others, basic mental abilities not dependent on information are essential. Questions which test these things may not appear as pertinent to the duties of the position as those which test for knowledge and information. Yet they are often highly important parts of a fair examination. For very general questions, it is almost impossible to help you direct your study efforts. What we can do is to point out some of the more common of these general abilities needed in public service positions and describe some typical questions.

1) General information

Broad, general information has been found useful for predicting job success in some kinds of work. This is tested in a variety of ways, from vocabulary lists to questions about current events. Basic background in some field of work, such as sociology or economics, may be sampled in a group of questions. Often these are principles which have become familiar to most persons through exposure rather than through formal training. It is difficult to advise you how to study for these questions; being alert to the world around you is our best suggestion.

2) Verbal ability

An example of an ability needed in many positions is verbal or language ability. Verbal ability is, in brief, the ability to use and understand words. Vocabulary and grammar tests are typical measures of this ability. Reading comprehension or paragraph interpretation questions are common in many kinds of civil service tests. You are given a paragraph of written material and asked to find its central meaning.

IV. KINDS OF QUESTIONS

1. Multiple-choice Questions

Most popular of the short-answer questions is the "multiple choice" or "best answer" question. It can be used, for example, to test for factual knowledge, ability to solve problems or judgment in meeting situations found at work.

A multiple-choice question is normally one of three types:
- It can begin with an incomplete statement followed by several possible endings. You are to find the one ending which best completes the statement, although some of the others may not be entirely wrong.
- It can also be a complete statement in the form of a question which is answered by choosing one of the statements listed.
- It can be in the form of a problem – again you select the best answer.

Here is an example of a multiple-choice question with a discussion which should give you some clues as to the method for choosing the right answer:

When an employee has a complaint about his assignment, the action which will best help him overcome his difficulty is to
- A. discuss his difficulty with his coworkers
- B. take the problem to the head of the organization
- C. take the problem to the person who gave him the assignment
- D. say nothing to anyone about his complaint

In answering this question, you should study each of the choices to find which is best. Consider choice "A" – Certainly an employee may discuss his complaint with fellow employees, but no change or improvement can result, and the complaint remains unresolved. Choice "B" is a poor choice since the head of the organization probably does not know what assignment you have been given, and taking your problem to him is known as "going over the head" of the supervisor. The supervisor, or person who made the assignment, is the person who can clarify it or correct any injustice. Choice "C" is, therefore, correct. To say nothing, as in choice "D," is unwise. Supervisors have and interest in knowing the problems employees are facing, and the employee is seeking a solution to his problem.

2. True/False

3. Matching Questions

Matching an answer from a column of choices within another column.

V. RECORDING YOUR ANSWERS

Computer terminals are used more and more today for many different kinds of exams.

For an examination with very few applicants, you may be told to record your answers in the test booklet itself. Separate answer sheets are much more common. If this separate answer sheet is to be scored by machine – and this is often the case – it is highly important that you mark your answers correctly in order to get credit.

VI. BEFORE THE TEST

YOUR PHYSICAL CONDITION IS IMPORTANT

If you are not well, you can't do your best work on tests. If you are half asleep, you can't do your best either. Here are some tips:

1) Get about the same amount of sleep you usually get. Don't stay up all night before the test, either partying or worrying—DON'T DO IT!
2) If you wear glasses, be sure to wear them when you go to take the test. This goes for hearing aids, too.
3) If you have any physical problems that may keep you from doing your best, be sure to tell the person giving the test. If you are sick or in poor health, you relay cannot do your best on any test. You can always come back and take the test some other time.

Common sense will help you find procedures to follow to get ready for an examination. Too many of us, however, overlook these sensible measures. Indeed, nervousness and fatigue have been found to be the most serious reasons why applicants fail to do their best on civil service tests. Here is a list of reminders:

- Begin your preparation early – Don't wait until the last minute to go scurrying around for books and materials or to find out what the position is all about.
- Prepare continuously – An hour a night for a week is better than an all-night cram session. This has been definitely established. What is more, a night a week for a month will return better dividends than crowding your study into a shorter period of time.
- Locate the place of the exam – You have been sent a notice telling you when and where to report for the examination. If the location is in a different town or otherwise unfamiliar to you, it would be well to inquire the best route and learn something about the building.
- Relax the night before the test – Allow your mind to rest. Do not study at all that night. Plan some mild recreation or diversion; then go to bed early and get a good night's sleep.
- Get up early enough to make a leisurely trip to the place for the test – This way unforeseen events, traffic snarls, unfamiliar buildings, etc. will not upset you.
- Dress comfortably – A written test is not a fashion show. You will be known by number and not by name, so wear something comfortable.
- Leave excess paraphernalia at home – Shopping bags and odd bundles will get in your way. You need bring only the items mentioned in the official notice you received; usually everything you need is provided. Do not bring reference books to the exam. They will only confuse those last minutes and be taken away from you when in the test room.

- Arrive somewhat ahead of time – If because of transportation schedules you must get there very early, bring a newspaper or magazine to take your mind off yourself while waiting.
- Locate the examination room – When you have found the proper room, you will be directed to the seat or part of the room where you will sit. Sometimes you are given a sheet of instructions to read while you are waiting. Do not fill out any forms until you are told to do so; just read them and be prepared.
- Relax and prepare to listen to the instructions
- If you have any physical problem that may keep you from doing your best, be sure to tell the test administrator. If you are sick or in poor health, you really cannot do your best on the exam. You can come back and take the test some other time.

VII. AT THE TEST

The day of the test is here and you have the test booklet in your hand. The temptation to get going is very strong. Caution! There is more to success than knowing the right answers. You must know how to identify your papers and understand variations in the type of short-answer question used in this particular examination. Follow these suggestions for maximum results from your efforts:

1) Cooperate with the monitor

The test administrator has a duty to create a situation in which you can be as much at ease as possible. He will give instructions, tell you when to begin, check to see that you are marking your answer sheet correctly, and so on. He is not there to guard you, although he will see that your competitors do not take unfair advantage. He wants to help you do your best.

2) Listen to all instructions

Don't jump the gun! Wait until you understand all directions. In most civil service tests you get more time than you need to answer the questions. So don't be in a hurry. Read each word of instructions until you clearly understand the meaning. Study the examples, listen to all announcements and follow directions. Ask questions if you do not understand what to do.

3) Identify your papers

Civil service exams are usually identified by number only. You will be assigned a number; you must not put your name on your test papers. Be sure to copy your number correctly. Since more than one exam may be given, copy your exact examination title.

4) Plan your time

Unless you are told that a test is a "speed" or "rate of work" test, speed itself is usually not important. Time enough to answer all the questions will be provided, but this does not mean that you have all day. An overall time limit has been set. Divide the total time (in minutes) by the number of questions to determine the approximate time you have for each question.

5) Do not linger over difficult questions

If you come across a difficult question, mark it with a paper clip (useful to have along) and come back to it when you have been through the booklet. One caution if you do this – be sure to skip a number on your answer sheet as well. Check often to be sure that you have not lost your place and that you are marking in the row numbered the same as the question you are answering.

6) Read the questions

Be sure you know what the question asks! Many capable people are unsuccessful because they failed to read the questions correctly.

7) Answer all questions

Unless you have been instructed that a penalty will be deducted for incorrect answers, it is better to guess than to omit a question.

8) Speed tests

It is often better NOT to guess on speed tests. It has been found that on timed tests people are tempted to spend the last few seconds before time is called in marking answers at random – without even reading them – in the hope of picking up a few extra points. To discourage this practice, the instructions may warn you that your score will be "corrected" for guessing. That is, a penalty will be applied. The incorrect answers will be deducted from the correct ones, or some other penalty formula will be used.

9) Review your answers

If you finish before time is called, go back to the questions you guessed or omitted to give them further thought. Review other answers if you have time.

10) Return your test materials

If you are ready to leave before others have finished or time is called, take ALL your materials to the monitor and leave quietly. Never take any test material with you. The monitor can discover whose papers are not complete, and taking a test booklet may be grounds for disqualification.

VIII. EXAMINATION TECHNIQUES

1) Read the general instructions carefully. These are usually printed on the first page of the exam booklet. As a rule, these instructions refer to the timing of the examination; the fact that you should not start work until the signal and must stop work at a signal, etc. If there are any special instructions, such as a choice of questions to be answered, make sure that you note this instruction carefully.

2) When you are ready to start work on the examination, that is as soon as the signal has been given, read the instructions to each question booklet, underline any key words or phrases, such as least, best, outline, describe and the like. In this way you will tend to answer as requested rather than discover on reviewing your paper that you listed without describing, that you selected the worst choice rather than the best choice, etc.

3) If the examination is of the objective or multiple-choice type – that is, each question will also give a series of possible answers: A, B, C or D, and you are called upon to select the best answer and write the letter next to that answer on your answer paper – it is advisable to start answering each question in turn. There may be anywhere from 50 to 100 such questions in the three or four hours allotted and you can see how much time would be taken if you read through all the questions before beginning to answer any. Furthermore, if you

come across a question or group of questions which you know would be difficult to answer, it would undoubtedly affect your handling of all the other questions.

4) If the examination is of the essay type and contains but a few questions, it is a moot point as to whether you should read all the questions before starting to answer any one. Of course, if you are given a choice – say five out of seven and the like – then it is essential to read all the questions so you can eliminate the two that are most difficult. If, however, you are asked to answer all the questions, there may be danger in trying to answer the easiest one first because you may find that you will spend too much time on it. The best technique is to answer the first question, then proceed to the second, etc.

5) Time your answers. Before the exam begins, write down the time it started, then add the time allowed for the examination and write down the time it must be completed, then divide the time available somewhat as follows:
   - If 3-1/2 hours are allowed, that would be 210 minutes. If you have 80 objective-type questions, that would be an average of 2-1/2 minutes per question. Allow yourself no more than 2 minutes per question, or a total of 160 minutes, which will permit about 50 minutes to review.
   - If for the time allotment of 210 minutes there are 7 essay questions to answer, that would average about 30 minutes a question. Give yourself only 25 minutes per question so that you have about 35 minutes to review.

6) The most important instruction is to read each question and make sure you know what is wanted. The second most important instruction is to time yourself properly so that you answer every question. The third most important instruction is to answer every question. Guess if you have to but include something for each question. Remember that you will receive no credit for a blank and will probably receive some credit if you write something in answer to an essay question. If you guess a letter – say "B" for a multiple-choice question – you may have guessed right. If you leave a blank as an answer to a multiple-choice question, the examiners may respect your feelings but it will not add a point to your score. Some exams may penalize you for wrong answers, so in such cases only, you may not want to guess unless you have some basis for your answer.

7) Suggestions
   a. Objective-type questions
      1. Examine the question booklet for proper sequence of pages and questions
      2. Read all instructions carefully
      3. Skip any question which seems too difficult; return to it after all other questions have been answered
      4. Apportion your time properly; do not spend too much time on any single question or group of questions
      5. Note and underline key words – all, most, fewest, least, best, worst, same, opposite, etc.
      6. Pay particular attention to negatives
      7. Note unusual option, e.g., unduly long, short, complex, different or similar in content to the body of the question
      8. Observe the use of "hedging" words – probably, may, most likely, etc.

9. Make sure that your answer is put next to the same number as the question
10. Do not second-guess unless you have good reason to believe the second answer is definitely more correct
11. Cross out original answer if you decide another answer is more accurate; do not erase until you are ready to hand your paper in
12. Answer all questions; guess unless instructed otherwise
13. Leave time for review

b. Essay questions
1. Read each question carefully
2. Determine exactly what is wanted. Underline key words or phrases.
3. Decide on outline or paragraph answer
4. Include many different points and elements unless asked to develop any one or two points or elements
5. Show impartiality by giving pros and cons unless directed to select one side only
6. Make and write down any assumptions you find necessary to answer the questions
7. Watch your English, grammar, punctuation and choice of words
8. Time your answers; don't crowd material

8) Answering the essay question

Most essay questions can be answered by framing the specific response around several key words or ideas. Here are a few such key words or ideas:

M's: manpower, materials, methods, money, management
P's: purpose, program, policy, plan, procedure, practice, problems, pitfalls, personnel, public relations

a. Six basic steps in handling problems:
1. Preliminary plan and background development
2. Collect information, data and facts
3. Analyze and interpret information, data and facts
4. Analyze and develop solutions as well as make recommendations
5. Prepare report and sell recommendations
6. Install recommendations and follow up effectiveness

b. Pitfalls to avoid
1. Taking things for granted – A statement of the situation does not necessarily imply that each of the elements is necessarily true; for example, a complaint may be invalid and biased so that all that can be taken for granted is that a complaint has been registered
2. Considering only one side of a situation – Wherever possible, indicate several alternatives and then point out the reasons you selected the best one
3. Failing to indicate follow up – Whenever your answer indicates action on your part, make certain that you will take proper follow-up action to see how successful your recommendations, procedures or actions turn out to be
4. Taking too long in answering any single question – Remember to time your answers properly

EXAMINATION SECTION

EXAMINATION SECTION
TEST 1

DIRECTIONS: Each question or incomplete statement is followed by several suggested answers or completions. Select the one that BEST answers the question or completes the statement. *PRINT THE LETTER OF THE CORRECT ANSWER IN THE SPACE AT THE RIGHT.*

1. Which of the following medication types is manufactured to prevent irritation to the stomach?
    A. Capsule B. Caplet
    C. Buffered tablet D. Emulsion
    1.____

2. Which of the following is a solid dosage form in which the drug is enclosed either in a hard or soft shell of soluble material?
    A. Capsule B. Caplet
    C. Tablet D. Buffered tablet
    2.____

3. A(n) _____ is a clear, sweetened, flavored, hydroalcoholic liquid medication intended for oral use.
    A. emulsion B. elixir
    C. fluid extract D. suspension
    3.____

4. _____ is a liquid preparation for external use, usually applied by friction to the skin.
    A. Ointment B. Cream C. Gel D. Liniment
    4.____

5. Which of the following is a very small pill, usually gelatin or sugar-coated, containing a drug to be given in a small dose?
    A. Gelcap B. Granule
    C. Enteric coated tablet D. Caplet
    5.____

6. Which of the following is an alcoholic solution prepared from vegetable materials or from chemical substances and commonly used as a skin disinfectant?
    A. Tincture B. Liniment C. Syrup D. Troche
    6.____

7. _____ is defined as the measurement of the rate of absorption and the total amount of drug that reaches the systemic circulation.
    A. Absorption B. Bioavailability
    C. Bio-transformation D. Metabolism
    7.____

8. Which of the following is a substance that is produced to alter actions of liver enzymes?
    A. Agonist B. Antagonist
    C. Anti-metabolite D. Metabolite
    8.____

9. A(n) _____ is a drug that produces a functional change in a cell.
   A. agonist
   B. antagonist
   C. anti-metabolite
   D. metabolite

9.____

10. Which of the following is defined as the conversion of a drug within the body, also referred to as metabolism?
    A. Absorption
    B. Bioavailability
    C. Bio-transformation
    D. Filtration

10.____

11. _____ is defined as the process of particles in a fluid moving from an area area of higher concentration to an area of lower concentration, thereby resulting in an even distribution of the particles in the fluid.
    A. Active transport
    B. Filtration
    C. Diffusion
    D. Tubular secretion

11.____

12. Which of the following is the MOST common and important mode of traversal of drugs through membranes?
    A. Active transport
    B. Passive transport
    C. Tubular secretion
    D. Re-absorption

12.____

13. _____ is defined as the study of the biochemical and physiological effects of drugs.
    A. Phamacodynamics
    B. Pharmacokinetics
    C. Toxicology
    D. Pharmacotherapy

13.____

14. _____ is defined as the study of absorption, distribution, metabolism, and excretion of drugs.
    A. Pharmacodynamics
    B. Pharmacokinetics
    C. Toxicolocy
    B. Pharmacotherapy

14.____

15. The process of drugs reaching the liver where they are partially metabolized prior to being through the body is referred to as
    A. filtration
    B. hepatic portal circulation
    C. dose effect relationship
    D. first pass effect

15.____

16. A unique, strange, or unpredicted reaction to a drug is known as
    A. hypersensitivity
    B. anaphylactic reaction
    C. idiosyncratic reaction
    D. serotonin syndrome

16.____

17. A severe, life-threatening, allergic reaction to a drug is known as
    A. hypersensitivity
    B. anaphylactic reaction
    C. idiosyncratic reaction
    D. serotonin syndrome

17.____

18. Which of the following is a neurotransmitter that plays a major role in cognitive function and memory formation as well as motor control?
    A. Acetylcholine
    B. Dopamine
    C. Serotonin
    D. Norepinephrine

18.____

19. Which of the following is an amino acid that acts like a neurotransmitter and is a key molecule in cellular metabolism, playing an important role in the body's disposal of excess or waste nitrogen?
    A. Gamma-aminobutyric acid
    B. Melatonin
    C. Dopamine
    D. Glutamate

20. _____ is defined as reduced responsiveness of a drug because of adaptation to a drug.
    A. Addiction
    B. Tolerance
    C. Polypharmacy
    D. Placebo

21. Which of the following is an important hormone secreted from the pineal gland that is believed to induce sleep?
    A. Melatonin
    B. Serotonin
    C. Dopamine
    D. Acetylcholine

22. Which of the following receptors mediate responses to acetylcholine?
    A. Adrenergic receptors
    B. Alpha receptors
    C. Beta receptors
    D. Cholinergic receptors

23. Epinephrine is a major neurotransmitter that is released by which of the following?
    A. Postganglionic neurons of the sympathetic nervous system
    B. Adrenal medulla
    C. Pineal gland
    D. Pituitary gland

24. Which of the following is a neurotransmitter that is naturally produced in the brain that affects motor control, memory, attention span, the ability to problem solve, motivation, pleasure, and creative thought?
    A. Acetylcholine
    B. Dopamine
    C. Serotonin
    D. Norepinephrine

25. Norepinephrine is a chemical neurotransmitter that is released by which of the following?
    A. Postganglionic neurons of the sympathetic nervous system
    B. Adrenal medulla
    C. Pineal gland
    D. Pituitary gland

KEY (CORRECT ANSWERS)

1. C
2. A
3. B
4. D
5. B

6. A
7. B
8. C
9. A
10. C

11. C
12. B
13. A
14. B
15. D

16. C
17. B
18. A
19. D
20. B

21. A
22. D
23. B
24. B
25. A

TEST 2

DIRECTIONS: Each question or incomplete statement is followed by several suggested answers or completions. Select the one that BEST answers the question or completes the statement. *PRINT THE LETTER OF THE CORRECT ANSWER IN THE SPACE AT THE RIGHT.*

1. Which of the following is defined as the amount of drug needed to produce a response?
   A. Tolerance   B. Potency   C. Efficacy   D. Duration

   1.____

2. _____ is defined as the maximum response of the drug regardless of the dose.
   A. Tolerance   B. Potency   C. Efficacy   D. Duration

   2.____

3. All of the following are positive effects of medications being administered orally EXCEPT
   A. safest
   B. least expensive
   C. most convenient
   D. small area of absorption

   3.____

4. Which route of drug administration has the MOST rapid drug response?
   A. Oral
   B. Rectal
   C. Transdermal
   D. Intravenous

   4.____

5. Through what route is insulin properly administered?
   A. Subcutaneous
   B. Intramuscular
   C. Intravenous
   D. Transdermal

   5.____

6. Through what route is a tuberculin skin test properly administered?
   A. Transdermal
   B. Intradermal
   C. Intramuscular
   D. Intravenous

   6.____

7. Absorption of oral medications occurs PRIMARILY in which of the following locations?
   A. Stomach
   B. Liver
   C. Small intestine
   D. Large intestine

   7.____

8. All of the following are criteria that will influence the drug levels and kinetics of drug exposure to the tissues and influence the performance and pharmacological activity of a drug EXCEPT
   A. absorption   B. secretion   C. metabolism   D. excretion

   8.____

9. When a medication is administered intravenously, which step is bypassed?
   A. Absorption   B. Distribution   C. Metabolism   D. Excretion

   9.____

10. In which area of the body does the majority of drug metabolism take place?
    A. Stomach
    B. Liver
    C. Small intestine
    D. Large intestine

    10.____

11. In which area of the body does the elimination of drugs occur?   11.____
    A. Stomach   B. Liver   C. Kidneys   D. Pancreas

12. Which of the following describes an adverse reaction that occurs when   12.____
    the desired effect is excessive?
    A. Anaphylactic reaction   B. Idiosyncratic reaction
    C. Toxic effect   D. Teratogenic effect

13. Which of the following describes an adverse drug reaction that occurs due   13.____
    to the casual relationship between the drug use of a mother causing congenital
    abnormalities?
    A. Anaphylactic reaction   B. Idiosyncratic reaction
    C. Toxic effect   D. Teratogenic effect

14. All of the following medications are used for the treatment of hypertension   14.____
    EXCEPT
    A. Timolol   B. Propranolol   C. Atenolol   D. Metoprolol

15. Which of the following types of medication stimulates bronchial glands to   15.____
    secrete water to make mucous easier to dislodge?
    A. Mucolytics   B. Expectorants
    C. Beractant   D. Surfactant

16. In which route of administration is first pass metabolism avoided?   16.____
    A. Oral   B. Respiratory
    C. Intramuscular   D. Intravenous

17. All of the following are advantages for topical administration of medication   17.____
    EXCEPT
    A. inexpensive   B. treats the affected site
    C. systemic absorption may occur   D. self-administered

18. All of the following are disadvantages of respiratory administration of   18.____
    medication EXCEPT
    A. expensive
    B. can be absorbed into systemic circulation
    C. high potential for abuse
    D. must have intranasal administration for optimum efficacy

19. All of the following are advantages to enteral administration of medication   19.____
    EXCEPT
    A. inexpensive   B. convenient
    C. safe   D. predictable absorption

20. In what area are sustained release products absorbed?   20.____
    A. Stomach   B. Liver   C. Kidneys   D. Colon

21. Which of the following is defined as fluid infusing into the tissues surrounding a venipuncture site causing swelling and redness?
    A. Infiltration
    B. Extravasation
    C. Infestation
    D. Localization

    21._____

22. Which of the following is defined as the infiltration of a vesicant or chemotherapy agent that can result in cellular damage?
    A. Manifestation
    B. Extravasation
    C. Infestation
    D. Localization

    22._____

23. All of the following medications can commonly be administered intra-articularly EXCEPT
    A. corticosteroids
    B. antimicrobials
    C. diuretics
    D. anesthetics

    23._____

24. If a medication is administered intrathecally, where is that medication administered?
    A. In a joint space
    B. Into a bone
    C. In a localized lesion
    D. Into the spinal canal

    24._____

25. What is the significance of a medication having a pregnancy category of "X"?
    A. Shows no risks
    B. Remote chance of fetal risk
    C. Benefits outweigh the risks
    D. Contraindicated

    25._____

KEY (CORRECT ANSWERS)

1.	B		11.	C
2.	C		12.	C
3.	D		13.	D
4.	D		14.	A
5.	A		15.	B
6.	B		16.	B
7.	C		17.	C
8.	B		18.	A
9.	A		19.	D
10.	B		20.	D

21.	A
22.	B
23.	C
24.	D
25.	D

EXAMINATION SECTION
TEST 1

DIRECTIONS: Each question or incomplete statement is followed by several suggested answers or completions. Select the one that BEST answers the question or completes the statement. *PRINT THE LETTER OF THE CORRECT ANSWER IN THE SPACE AT THE RIGHT.*

1. Which piece of legislation required that "secret elixirs" containing ingredients such as cocaine, heroin, morphine, and alcohol be labeled with correct information about their ingredients as well as suggested dosages?
    A. Federal Food and Drug Act of 1906
    B. Narcotic Tax Act of 1914
    C. Durham Humphrey Amendment of 1951
    D. Kefauver-Harris Amendment of 1962

1._____

2. Which piece of legislation gave the Food and Drug Administration authority to require adequate testing of new drugs for safety?
    A. Federal Food and Drug Act of 1906
    B. Federal Food, Drug, and Cosmetic Act of 1938
    C. Poison Prevention Packaging Act of 1970
    D. Federal Privacy Act of 1974

2._____

3. The _____ Act provides authority for the Internal Revenue Service to collect tax on opiates through tax stamps.
    A. Harrison Narcotic   B. Controlled Substances
    C. Poison Prevention Packaging   D. Orphan Drug

3._____

4. Which of the following created a distinction between over-the-counter and legend drugs?
    A. Harrison Narcotic Act
    B. Controlled Substances Act
    C. The Durham Humphrey Amendment of 1951
    D. The Kefauver-Harris Amendment of 1962

4._____

5. Which of the following, also known as the "Drug Efficacy Amendment" requires drug manufacturers to provide proof of the effectiveness and safety of their drugs prior to approval?
    A. Federal Food and Drug Act of 1906
    B. Narcotic Tax Act of 1914
    C. Durham Humphrey Amendment of 1951
    D. Kefauver-Harris Amendment of 1962

5._____

6. Which federal agency merged into the Drug Enforcement Administration in 1973?
   A. Environmental Protection Agency
   B. Food and Drug Administration
   C. Department of Transportation
   D. Bureau of Narcotics and Dangerous Drugs

7. Which piece of legislation completed replaced the Harrison Narcotic Act requires comprehensive record keeping and transaction tracking, and is enforced by the Drug Enforcement Agency under the U.S. Department of Justice?
   A. Drug Abuse Prevention/Control Act of 1970
   B. Poison Prevention Packaging Act of 1970
   C. Combat Methamphetamine Epidemic Act
   D. Drug Listing Act of 1972

8. Which piece of legislation is designed to reduce the risk of children ingesting dangerous substances and requires locking caps on most prescriptions?
   A. Drug Abuse Prevention/Control Act of 1970
   B. Poison Prevention Packaging Act of 1970
   C. Drug Listing Act of 1972
   D. Orphan Drug Act of 1983

9. According to the Combat Methamphetamine Act of 2005, what is the 30-day purchase limit for over-the-counter products containing pseudoephedrine?
   A. 3.6 grams   B. 5.8 grams   C. 7.5 grams   D. 9.0 grams

10. Which piece of legislation created the 11 digit national drug code?
    A. Drug Listing Act of 1972
    B. The Federal Privacy Act of 1974
    C. Orphan Drug Act of 1983
    D. Prescription Drug Marketing Act of 1987

11. The _____ limited information in which the federal government can access.
    A. Drug Listing Act of 1972
    B. Federal Privacy Act of 1974
    C. Orphan Drug Act of 1983
    D. Prescription Drug Marketing Act of 1987

12. The _____ provides a tax incentive for manufacturers to develop medications to treat life-threatening or debilitating rare diseases.
    A. Drug Listing Act of 1972
    B. Federal Privacy Act of 1974
    C. Orphan Drug Act of 1983
    D. Prescription Drug Marketing Act of 1987

13. Which piece of legislation encouraged the creation of generic drugs by stream-   13.____
lining the process for generic drug approval and extending patent licenses?
    A. Hatch-Waxman Act
    B. Prescription Drug Marketing Act
    C. Omnibus Budget Reconciliation Act
    D. Orphan Drug Act

14. Which of the following prohibits reimportation of drugs and forbids the   14.____
sale of samples?
    A. Hatch-Waxman Act
    B. Prescription Drug Marketing Act
    C. Omnibus Budget Reconciliation Act
    D. Orphan Drug Act

15. The _____ revised Medicare and Medicaid conditions of participation   15.____
regarding long-term care facilities and pharmacies.
    A. Omnibus Budget Reconciliation Act of 1987
    B. The Anabolic Steroid Control Act of 1990
    C. Food and Drug Administration Safe Medical Devices Act of 1990
    D. Health Insurance Portability and Accountability Act of 1996

16. The Anabolic Steroid Control Act of 1990 was designed to implement   16.____
harsher penalties on which type of steroid abusers?
    A. Physicians   B. Administrators
    C. Athletes   D. Terminally ill

17. Which piece of legislation was urged by 107 accidental deaths caused by   17.____
anti-freeze, diethylene glycol, poisoning?
    A. Federal Food and Drug Act of 1906
    B. Federal Food, Drug, and Cosmetic Act of 1938
    C. Poison Prevention Packaging Act of 1970
    D. Federal Privacy Act of 1974

18. The _____ Act draws the distinction between compounding and manufacturing.   18.____
    A. FDA Modernization   B. Prescription Drug Marketing
    C. Hatch-Waxman Amendment   D. Orphan Drug Act

19. Which government agency regulates advertising of over-the-counter   19.____
medication?
    A. Food and Drug Administration
    B. Federal Trade Commission
    C. Environmental Protection Agency
    D. Federal Communications Commission

20. Which governmental agency regulates the advertising of legend drugs?   20.____
    A. Food and Drug Administration
    B. Federal Trade Commission
    C. Environmental Protection Agency
    D. Federal Communications Commission

21. Which form should a pharmacy use to apply for registration by the Drug Enforcement Agency?
    A. DEA 224 B. DEA 224b C. DEA 510 D. DEA 41

22. What form should a pharmacy use to notify the Drug Enforcement Agency of breakage and spillage of controlled substances?
    A. DEA 41 B. DEA 106 C. DEA 224 D. DEA 510

23. What form should a pharmacy use to notify the Drug Enforcement Agency of theft or loss of controlled substances?
    A. DEA 41 B. DEA 106 C. DEA 224 D. DEA 510

24. For what time period should a pharmacy retain all records regarding Schedule-III through Schedule-V controlled substances?
    A. 1 year B. 2 years C. 5 years D. 7 years

25. All of the following are required by the Drug Enforcement Agency on a prescription for controlled substances EXCEPT
    A. physician's full name and address
    B. DEA registration number
    C. quantity prescribed
    D. expiration date

KEY (CORRECT ANSWERS)

1.	A		11.	B
2.	B		12.	C
3.	A		13.	A
4.	C		14.	B
5.	D		15.	A
6.	D		16.	C
7.	A		17.	B
8.	B		18.	A
9.	D		19.	B
10.	A		20.	A

21. A
22. A
23. B
24. B
25. D

TEST 2

DIRECTIONS: Each question or incomplete statement is followed by several suggested answers or completions. Select the one that BEST answers the question or completes the statement. *PRINT THE LETTER OF THE CORRECT ANSWER IN THE SPACE AT THE RIGHT.*

1. Which form should be used in order to legally prescribe and dispense methadone?
   A. DEA 41 B. DEA 106 C. DEA 363 D. DEA 510

   1.____

2. How long after occurrence should loss or theft of schedule listed chemical products be reported?
   A. 24 hours B. 48 hours C. 7 days D. 15 days

   2.____

3. Schedule-_____ is a class of drugs that have no accepted medical use in the U.S. and have a very high abuse potential.
   A. I B. II C. III D. IV

   3.____

4. Schedule-_____ is a class of drugs that has a high potential for abuse but is used for medicinal purposes and may lead to severe psychological or physical dependence.
   A. I B. II C. III D. IV

   4.____

5. What is the MAXIMUM number of refills allowed for a Schedule-III through Schedule-V medication in a six-month period?
   A. 0 B. 1 C. 3 D. 5

   5.____

6. There are zero refills permitted for a Schedule-_____ class of medications.
   A. I B. II C. III D. IV

   6.____

7. Which governmental agency provides guidance on storage requirements and what to do in case of spill or contact with eyes?
   A. Joint Commission
   B. Department of Health
   C. Occupational Safety and Health Administration
   D. Environmental Protection Agency

   7.____

8. The mission of which agency is to improve the safety and quality of care within healthcare facilities?
   A. Joint Commission
   B. Department of Health
   C. Occupational Safety and Health Administration
   D. Environmental Protection Agency

   8.____

9. Schedule-_____ is a class of medication that CANNOT be prescribed by a physician.
   A. I B. II C. III D. IV

   9.____

10. Which of the following medications may be dispensed without a childproof cap?
    A. Vicodin
    B. Lorazepam
    C. Nitroglycerin
    D. Percocet

11. _____ is defined as the mishandling of medications that can lead to contamination.
    A. Adulteration
    B. Misbranding
    C. Compounding
    D. Encryption

12. Which piece of legislation requires pharmacists to offer counseling to Medicaid patients regarding medications?
    A. 1990 Omnibus Budget Reconciliation Act
    B. 1996 Health Insurance Portability and Accountability Act
    C. 2003 Medicare Modernization Act
    D. 2010 Patient Protection and Affordable Care Act

13. The _____ defined the scope of health information that may or may not be shared among healthcare providers without patient consent and provided for broad and stringent regulations to protect patients' right to privacy.
    A. 1990 Omnibus Budget Reconciliation Act
    B. 1996 Health Insurance Portability and Accountability Act
    C. 2003 Medicare Modernization Act
    D. 2010 Patient Protection and Affordable Care Act

14. The _____ established optional Medicare Part D to provide coverage for prescription drugs and medication therapy management.
    A. 1990 Omnibus Budget Reconciliation Act
    B. 1996 Health Insurance Portability and Accountability Act
    C. 2003 Medicare Modernization Act
    D. 2010 Patient Protection and Affordable Care Act

15. Which piece of legislation established user fees to enhance access to medication and medical devices and made provisions for addressing drug product shortages in the United States?
    A. 2003 Medicare Modernization Act
    B. 2005 Combat Methamphetamine Epidemic Act
    C. 2010 Patient Protection and Affordable Care Act
    D. 2012 FDA Safety and Innovation Act

16. How many patients are typically included in Phase 1 of human drug testing?
    A. 1-20
    B. 20-100
    C. Several hundred
    D. Several thousand

17. What is the PRIMARY purpose of Phase 1 human drug testing?
    A. Safety
    B. Efficacy
    C. Dosage
    D. Tolerance

3 (#2)

18. Phase 2 human drug testing typically lasts for what time period? 18.____
    A. Several months B. Several months – 2 years
    C. 1 year – 4 years D. 3 years – 5 years

19. What is the PRIMARY purpose of Phase 21 human drug testing? 19.____
    A. Safety B. Efficacy C. Dosage D. Tolerance

20. All of the following are purposes for Phase 3 human drug testing EXCEPT 20.____
    A. safety B. efficacy C. dosage D. tolerance

21. For what time period must records be kept for C-II controlled substances? 21.____
    A. 1 year B. 3 years C. 5 years D. 7 years

22. Which piece of legislation prohibited false claims about the therapeutic effect of a drug? 22.____
    A. Sherley Amendment of 1911
    B. Narcotic Tax Act of 1914
    C. Durham Humphrey Amendment of 1951
    D. Kefauver-Harris Amendment of 1962

23. What is the prescription expiration date of a legend drug? 23.____
    A. 4 months B. 6 months C. 9 months D. 12 months

24. What is the prescription expiration date of a controlled substance? 24.____
    A. 30 days B. 60 days C. 90 days D. 6 months

25. All of the following are exceptions to the Poison Prevention Packaging Act of 1970 EXCEPT 25.____
    A. asthmatic patients
    B. emergency medications
    C. requests written from patient/prescriber
    D. labeled as non-childproof on over-the-counter products

KEY (CORRECT ANSWERS)

1.	C	11.	A
2.	D	12.	A
3.	A	13.	B
4.	B	14.	C
5.	D	15.	D
6.	B	16.	B
7.	C	17.	A
8.	A	18.	B
9.	A	19.	B
10.	C	20.	D

21.	D
22.	A
23.	D
24.	D
25.	A

TEST 3

DIRECTIONS: Each question or incomplete statement is followed by several suggested answers or completions. Select the one that BEST answers the question or completes the statement. *PRINT THE LETTER OF THE CORRECT ANSWER IN THE SPACE AT THE RIGHT.*

1. The state or federal law that prohibits the administration of a drug to any person other than the person to whom it was prescribed is known as _____ warning.
    A. black box
    B. transfer
    C. substitution
    D. administration

    1._____

2. All of the following are safety considerations all pharmacies must have EXCEPT
    A. the number of poison control center in dispensing area
    B. reference guide to toxicities of ingestion or topical exposure
    C. MSDS sheets for hazardous materials
    D. antidotes for all potentially toxic medications

    2._____

3. For what time period must a poison log be kept?
    A. 1 year   B. 3 years   C. 5 years   D. 7 years

    3._____

4. A poison log must include all of the following after a sale EXCEPT
    A. date of purchase
    B. potential health hazards of product
    C. name and quantity of product
    D. reason for purchase

    4._____

5. All poisonous substance labels must include all of the following EXCEPT
    A. the word **POISON** boldly printed
    B. complete name of the poison
    C. directions for use
    D. potential health hazards

    5._____

6. The _____ book lists all sources of drug products groups as pharmaceutical equivalents.
    A. Black   B. Blue   C. Yellow   D. Orange

    6._____

7. Which reference source includes selected laws and regulations for controlled substances?
    A. Physician's Desk Reference
    B. USP DI Volume I
    C. USP DI Volume II
    D. USP DI Volume III

    7._____

8. The statement "Rx Only" is required to appear on the packages of all of the following EXCEPT
    A. legend drugs
    B. orphan drugs
    C. controlled substances
    D. over-the-counter medications

    8._____

17

9. A pharmacist can refuse to fill a prescription in which of the following situations?
   A. The quantity of the controlled drug has been changed.
   B. Patient is unknown to the pharmacist.
   C. Patient has a history of illicit drug abuse.
   D. The prescribing physician is from another city.

10. Which of the following BEST describes the use of an FDA approved medication for a use that is not FDA approved?
    A. Illegal   B. Off-label   C. Terminal   D. Orphan

11. The Marketing Act of 1987 guarantees that a company which discovers, patents, and develops a new drug has exclusive marketing rights for a time period of
    A. 10 years   B. 20 years   C. 50 years   D. forever

12. For what reason are certain drug products exempt from the requirement therapeutic equivalence?
    A. The grandfather clause   B. Their use in chemotherapy
    C. Their high therapeutic index   D. High levels of toxicity

13. Which of the following medications does NOT fall into the category of grandfathered drugs?
    A. Ephedrine   B. Epinephrine
    C. Phenobarbital   D. Ampicillin

14. The National Drug Code (NDC) consists of a series of
    A. letters only   B. letter and numbers
    C. numbers only   D. numbers and symbols

15. How often should hospital inpatients receiving oral estrogen therapy receive patient package inserts?
    A. Only at the first dose
    B. With the first dose and at the time of discharge
    C. Every 7 days
    D. Every 30 days

16. In order for a patient to be admitted to a comprehensive maintenance program, the patient must be physiologically dependent on narcotics for a minimum of
    A. 90 days   B. 180 days   C. 12 months   D. 18 months

17. According to the Omnibus Budget Reconciliation Act of 1990, who is responsible for performing retrospective drug utilization reviews?
    A. Each state
    B. All dispensing pharmacists
    C. Individual community pharmacies
    D. Hospital pharmacies

18. Which of the following BEST describes a "listed chemical"?
    A. A controlled substance
    B. A chemical used in manufacturing a controlled substance
    C. A chemical listed in the USP/NF
    D. A chemical listed in the USP DI

    18.____

19. Which person maintains the authority for determining the schedule for a potentially new controlled substance?
    A. Director of the FDA
    B. Director of the DEA
    C. Attorney General of the United States
    D. Director of Health and Human Services

    19.____

20. The NDC number on a pharmaceutical package is divided into how many segments?
    A. 2   B. 3   C. 4   D. 5

    20.____

21. What number is given to the clinical trial phase that consists of post-marketing surveillance of a new drug that was recently introduced to the market?
    A. 2   B. 3   C. 4   D. 5

    21.____

22. A drug product consisting of tablets may be considered adulterated for all of the following reasons EXCEPT:
    A. Active drug has undergone partial decomposition
    B. Product contains an unapproved color additive
    C. Product does not indicate the number of tablets present
    D. Inactive ingredient has undergone partial decomposition

    22.____

23. The presence of which of the following additives in a commercial drug product requires a special label warning?
    A. Antioxidants   B. Tartrazine
    C. Sodium Benzoate   D. Artificial flavors

    23.____

24. If two generic companies manufacture a specific drug in several dosage forms, which dosage form is MOST likely to present problems with bioequivalence?
    A. Aerosol   B. Capsule   C. Tablet   D. Oral solution

    24.____

25. Which of the following is the appropriate format for the listing of ingredients on a product label?
    A. Additives and active ingredients are intermixed but listed alphabetically.
    B. Additives and active ingredients are intermixed and ranked by decreasing concentration.
    C. Additives and active ingredients are intermixed and ranked by increasing concentration.
    D. Additives are listed separately from the active ingredients.

    25.____

KEY (CORRECT ANSWERS)

1.	B		11.	B
2.	D		12.	A
3.	C		13.	D
4.	B		14.	C
5.	D		15.	D
6.	D		16.	C
7.	D		17.	A
8.	D		18.	B
9.	A		19.	C
10.	B		20.	B

21. C
22. C
23. B
24. A
25. D

TEST 4

DIRECTIONS: Each question or incomplete statement is followed by several suggested answers or completions. Select the one that BEST answers the question or completes the statement. *PRINT THE LETTER OF THE CORRECT ANSWER IN THE SPACE AT THE RIGHT.*

1. Which of the following information must be included on the barcode of drug products being sold to hospitals?
   A. NDC numbers
   B. DEA numbers
   C. Lot numbers
   D. Expiration dates

   1.____

2. Which person is authorized to designate the official name of a new drug?
   A. Director of the FDA
   B. Director of the DEA
   C. Attorney General of the United States
   D. Director of Health and Human Services

   2.____

3. What is the MAXIMUM volume of Ipecac Syrup that can be sold without a prescription?
   A. 15 ml   B. 30 ml   C. 45 ml   D. 60 ml

   3.____

4. What is the ONLY manner in which patients treated in an ambulatory care comprehensive narcotic treatment program can receive methadone doses?
   A. Orally
   B. Subcutaneously
   C. Intramuscularly
   D. Intravenously

   4.____

5. Which of the following is the total number of digits in the NDC number that may be present on a pharmaceutical package?
   A. 5-6   B. 8-9   C. 10-11   D. 15-16

   5.____

6. Which of the following is represented by the first series of digits in the NDC number of a drug product?
   A. Manufacturer
   B. Drug name
   C. Drug strength
   D. Therapeutic use

   6.____

7. Under which of the following conditions can practitioners of Traditional Chinese Medicine sell products containing ephedra?
   A. Ephedra concentration must be less than 1 mg/dose.
   B. Product may only be sold in a 10-day supply.
   C. A prescription must be issued for the product.
   D. Label does not indicate that the product is a dietary supplement.

   7.____

8. Which of the following must be present on the labels of nonprescription drug products intended for oral use?
   A. Sodium content of the active ingredients
   B. Sodium chloride content of the active ingredients
   C. Total sodium content of both active and inactive ingredients
   D. Total sodium chloride content of both active and inactive ingredients

   8.____

9. The term "donut hole" refers to a component of which of the following pieces of legislation?
   A. Prescription Drug Marketing Act of 1987
   B. Poison Prevention Act
   C. Medicare Part B
   D. Medicare Part D

10. The label of a parenteral product is NOT required to list the presence of
    A. antioxidants
    B. chelating agents
    C. inert gases
    D. antimicrobial preservatives

11. All of the following are mandatory on the labels of over-the-counter products EXCEPT
    A. NDC number
    B. name of manufacturer
    C. address of manufacturer
    D. adequate directions for use

12. All of the following are required on a label of a unit dose package prepared in a hospital EXCEPT
    A. beyond-use expiration date
    B. control number
    C. strength of drug
    D. manufacturer's expiration date

13. Which of the following statements is TRUE regarding grandfathered drugs?
    A. Can only be prescribed by generic name
    B. Found in the Orange Book as Code A only
    C. Found in the Orange Book as Code B only
    D. Often not listed in the Orange Book

14. What permanent identification must a pharmacy possess if it plans to electronically bill Medicare or Medicaid for prescriptions?
    A. FDA registration number
    B. DEA number
    C. NDC
    D. NPI

15. Which of the following statements is TRUE regarding samples of prescription drugs received from pharmaceutical companies?
    A. Can be sold through community pharmacies
    B. Can be given to patients by the prescriber
    C. Can be traded to another pharmacy for drugs
    D. Can be dispensed from a hospital pharmacy for inpatients

16. Which form must a pharmacy use in order to acquire grain alcohol for compounding?
    A. FDA 23A   B. ATF 11   C. ATF 222   D. DEA 222

17. Under which circumstance is an institution permitted to incorporate therapeutic substitution?
    A. If the institution obtains the proper license
    B. If the institution is supervised by a PharmD graduate
    C. If the institution is using a formulary system
    D. If it is a nonprofit institution

18. All of the following would be considered misbranding EXCEPT:
    A. The level of alcohol in the product is 5% V/V but the label states 15% V/V
    B. The names of inactive ingredients are not on the label
    C. The original bottle of 60 only contains 50 tablets
    D. One of the active drugs in a product is not identified on the label

19. Which of the following dosage forms is LEAST likely to present issues with bioequivalence?
    A. Transdermal patch
    B. IV solution
    C. Capsule
    D. Tablet

20. A statement that an over-the-counter product has a tamper evident feature may be placed on any of the following locations EXCEPT
    A. front of the package
    B. back of the package
    C. on the tamper evident device
    D. under the product name

21. A pharmacy that compounds large numbers of prescriptions may be cited by the FDA is the number of prescriptions being sent out-of-state exceeds what percentage?
    A. 5%
    B. 10%
    C. 25%
    D. 40%

22. The iPLEDGE program is intended to assure the appropriate and safe dispensing of which of the following medications?
    A. Thalidomide
    B. Neviraprine
    C. Isotretinoin
    D. Sildenafil

23. Which of the following must be imprinted on each commercial oral tablet?
    A. Company name
    B. Name and strength of the drug
    C. An expiration date
    D. A code identifying the company name, name of drug, strength of drug, date of manufacturing, and expiration date

24. Proposed regulations from the FDA are first published in which publication?
    A. Congressional Record
    B. Federal Register
    C. New York Times
    D. Wall Street Journal

25. For which medication must a patient sign an informed consent prior to receiving an original prescription?
    A. Isotretinoin
    B. Morphine Sulfate
    C. Sumatriptan
    D. Paroxetine

KEY (CORRECT ANSWERS)

1. A
2. D
3. B
4. A
5. C

6. A
7. D
8. C
9. D
10. C

11. A
12. D
13. D
14. D
15. B

16. B
17. C
18. A
19. B
20. C

21. A
22. C
23. D
24. B
25. A

EXAMINATION SECTION
TEST 1

DIRECTIONS: Each question or incomplete statement is followed by several suggested answers or completions. Select the one that BEST answers the question or completes the statement. *PRINT THE LETTER OF THE CORRECT ANSWER IN THE SPACE AT THE RIGHT.*

1. _____ is defined as the removal of pathogens to reduce transfer of microorganisms by cleaning any body part or surface that has been exposed to them.
   A. Surgical asepsis   B. Medical asepsis
   C. Sanitation   D. Disinfection

   1._____

2. Which of the following is defined as the destruction of all microorganisms, pathogenic, and non-pathogenic?
   A. Surgical asepsis   B. Medical asepsis
   C. Sanitation   D. Disinfection

   2._____

3. _____ is the process of killing or destroying all microorganisms and their pathogenic products.
   A. Sanitation   B. Disinfection
   C. Sterilization   D. Decontamination

   3._____

4. What type of airflow hood should be used for the preparation of numerous types of parenteral medications and sterile produce mixtures?
   A. Horizontal   B. Vertical   C. Diagonal   D. Negative

   4._____

5. What type of airflow hood should be used for all chemotherapeutic agents and can also be used to mix non-therapeutic agents?
   A. Horizontal   B. Vertical   C. Diagonal   D. Negative

   5._____

6. For what time period can sterile products be frozen?
   A. 10 days   B. 25 days   C. 30 days   D. 45 days

   6._____

7. At minimum, how often should laminar airflow workbenches be tested?
   A. Weekly   B. Monthly   C. Quarterly   D. Biannually

   7._____

8. If a laminar airflow workbench is turned off between aseptic processing sessions, for what time period should it run prior to being used again?
   A. 10 minutes   B. 20 minutes   C. 30 minutes   D. 40 minutes

   8._____

9. Which of the following pieces of personal protective equipment can be re-worn as long as it was properly stored in the anteroom?
   A. Gloves   B. Masks
   C. Gowns   D. Shoe coverings

   9._____

10. How often must training be conducted for personnel performing high-risk level compounding?
    A. Monthly   B. Quarterly   C. Biannually   D. Annually

11. Once a multi-dose vial has been opened, the beyond-use date must not exceed what time period unless otherwise referenced in the package insert?
    A. 7 days   B. 14 days   C. 21 days   D. 28 days

12. At what point should the rubber stopper on a vial be cleaned with a sterile alcohol wipe?
    A. Prior to beginning any point of the sterile compounding process
    B. Prior to placing the vial into the laminar flow workbench
    C. Immediately upon placing the vial into the laminar flow workbench
    D. Immediately prior to entering the port with a needle

13. At what distance from the outer edge of a laminar airflow workbench should all aseptic manipulations be made?
    A. 2 inches   B. 4 inches   C. 6 inches   D. 8 inches

14. Which of the following would be considered to be a multi-dose container?
    A. Syringe
    B. Ampule
    C. 50 ml preservative-free vial
    D. 20 ml vial containing benzyl alcohol

15. Which of the following statements is TRUE regarding sterile needles?
    A. Should be wiped with alcohol prior to use
    B. May be handled with sterile gloves
    C. Can be used repeatedly if remains in sterile environment
    D. Should remain in sterile packing until needed for use

16. Which of the following statements is TRUE regarding opening an ampule?
    A. Should be opened methodically to prevent excessive glass shards.
    B. Should be opened with extreme pressure to ensure a clean break.
    C. Neck of the ampule should be cleaned with an alcohol wipe and the wipe should remain in place to avoid accidental injury.
    D. Should be opened toward the HEPA filter to catch any loose shards of glass.

17. A filter needle is effective for removing which of the following?
    A. Fungi   B. Bacteria   C. Pyrogens   D. Particles

18. Where should the process of cleaning the laminar airflow workbench begin?
    A. The opening of the workbench and wipe toward the innermost surface in a sweeping side-to-side motion
    B. The opening of the workbench and wipe toward the innermost surface in a uniform line of movement
    C. The innermost surface and wipe toward the opening of the workbench in a uniform line of movement
    D. The innermost surface and wipe toward the opening of the workbench in a sweeping side-to-side motion

19. Through which method should the diluent be injected when reconstituting a drug?
    A. Rapidly into the vial and vigorously shaken
    B. Rapidly into the vial and then placed in the hood
    C. Slowly into the vial and then manually rotated
    D. Slowly into the vial and then placed in the hood

20. In which type of laminar flow workbench should all aseptic manipulations be carried out?
    A. ISO Class 5   B. ISO Class 6   C. ISO Class 7   D. ISO Class 8

21. The compounding of a parenteral nutrition is included under _____-risk sterile compounding.
    A. low   B. medium   C. high   D. critical

22. In the absence of passing a sterility test, the storage period for medium-risk preparations cannot exceed what time period prior to administration?
    A. 24 hours refrigerated   B. 72 hours refrigerated
    C. 9 days refrigerated   D. 14 days refrigerated

23. An immediate-use compounded sterile product is under a _____-risk level.
    A. low   B. medium   C. high   D. critical

24. For what time period can a single-dose vial exposed to ISO Class 5 air be used after initial needle puncture?
    A. 2 hours   B. 4 hours   C. 6 hours   D. 8 hours

25. For operations that prepare large volumes of hazardous drugs, how often should environmental sampling to detect uncontained hazardous drugs be performed?
    A. Weekly   B. Quarterly   C. Biannually   D. Annually

KEY (CORRECT ANSWERS)

1.	B		11.	D
2.	A		12.	D
3.	C		13.	C
4.	A		14.	D
5.	B		15.	D
6.	D		16.	C
7.	D		17.	D
8.	C		18.	C
9.	C		19.	A
10.	C		20.	A

21. B
22. C
23. B
24. C
25. C

TEST 2

DIRECTIONS: Each question or incomplete statement is followed by several suggested answers or completions. Select the one that BEST answers the question or completes the statement. *PRINT THE LETTER OF THE CORRECT ANSWER IN THE SPACE AT THE RIGHT.*

1. How often should the pressure differential between the buffer and ante-area and the pressure between the ante-area and general environment be reviewed and documented on a log sheet?
   A. Hourly   B. Every shift   C. Daily   D. Weekly

   1.____

2. Which of the following is the PREFERRED method for volumetric air sampling?
   A. Swabbing
   B. Electronic collection
   C. Impaction
   D. Settling plates

   2.____

3. Under what category would the measuring and mixing sterile ingredients in non-sterile devices prior to sterilization being performed be included?
   A. Low risk   B. Medium risk   C. High risk   D. Critical risk

   3.____

4. Which of the following is the PREFERRED method to terminally sterilize aqueous preparations that have been verified to maintain their full chemical and physical stability under the conditions employed?
   A. Irradiation   B. Dry heat   C. Filtration   D. Autoclave

   4.____

5. The buffer or clean room area which houses the laminar airflow workbench must provide air quality of at least ISO Class
   A. 5   B. 6   C. 7   D. 8

   5.____

6. Risk levels of compounded sterile products are assigned according to
   A. chemical stability
   B. storage conditions
   C. probability of contamination
   D. beyond use dating

   6.____

7. In the absence of a sterility test, what is the MAXIMUM beyond-use date for a high-risk compounded sterile preparation?
   A. 12 hours refrigerated
   B. 24 hours refrigerated
   C. 48 hours refrigerated
   D. 72 hours refrigerated

   7.____

8. Pushing a non-sterile solution through what size filter will sterilize the solution?
   A. 0.22μ   B. 0.4μ   C. 1.2μ   D. 5μ

   8.____

9. Which of the following is the PREFERRED method for terminal sterilization of an anhydrous high-risk level preparation?
   A. Radiation   B. Filtering   C. Autoclaving   D. Dry heat

   9.____

10. Which of the following statements is TRUE regarding barrier isolators?
    A. Should be placed in a buffer area away from open doors or high traffic areas
    B. May be placed in the ante-area
    C. Must be located in an ISO Class 8 clean room
    D. Should only be used for high-risk and hazardous sterile compounding

11. Which of the following is the PREFERRED method for sterility testing of high-risk sterile preparations?
    A. Membrane filtration
    B. Direct inoculation of culture medium
    C. TLC
    D. HPLC

12. At what point should gloved fingertip sampling be performed?
    A. Immediately following the compounding and sterilization of a high-risk level compounded sterile preparation
    B. Immediately following hand hygiene and garbing procedure
    C. Weekly for high-risk level compounding personnel
    D. Annually for high-risk level compounding personnel

13. A 5μ filter needle should be used when withdrawing a solution from a(n)
    A. ampule   B. vial   C. glass bottle   D. PVC bag

14. Which of the following statements is TRUE regarding the use of a laminar airflow workbench?
    A. Should be turned off between shifts for proper cleaning
    B. Should be turned off when not in use to conserve the HEPA filter
    C. Should be turned off at the end of every day
    D. Should operate continuously

15. With what product should antiseptic hand-cleansing be performed once inside the buffer area and before putting on sterile powder-free gloves?
    A. Alcohol-based surgical hand scrub
    B. Dakin's solution
    C. Hydrogen peroxide based gel
    D. Chlorhexidene scrub

16. Which volume of syringe would be MOST accurate for withdrawing 3.1 ml of solution?
    A. 3 ml   B. 5 ml   C. 10 ml   D. 20 ml

17. Which part(s) of the syringe cannot be touched in order to protect the integrity of sterilization?
    A. Tip and barrel   B. Plunger and barrel
    C. Tip and the plunger   D. Tip only

18. The interior working surfaces of the laminar airflow workbench should be cleaned with sterile 70% isopropyl alcohol and a
    A. sterile sponge
    B. sterile gauze pad
    C. clean paper towel
    D. clean, lint-free non-shedding cloth

19. Which of the following is the critical area within the ISO Class 5 primary engineering control where critical sites are exposed to unidirectional HEPA-filtered air?
    A. Direct compounding area
    B. Buffer area
    C. Pre-filter area
    D. Controlled area

20. Which of the following is the MOST common method of contaminating a compounded sterile preparation?
    A. Human touch
    B. Coring the rubber stopper
    C. Lint from the alcohol swab
    D. Repeated use of a needle

21. Prior to initiation of sterile compounding, you should vigorously scrub hands, nails, wrists, and forearms for at least 30 seconds with
    A. povidone-iodine
    B. 70% isopropyl alcohol
    C. hydrogen peroxide
    D. soap and warm water

22. Which of the following statements is TRUE regarding the use of an opened single-dose ampule?
    A. Cannot be stored for any time period
    B. Cannot be stored in excess of 1 hour
    C. Cannot be stored in excess of 4 hours
    D. Cannot be stored in excess of 8 hours

23. Which of the following statements is TRUE regarding withdrawing fluid from a vial?
    The volume of fluid should
    A. always be replaced with an equal volume of air
    B. be replaced with an equal volume of air except with hazardous or gas-producing drugs
    C. never be replaced with an equal volume of air
    D. be replaced with an equal volume of air with hazardous drugs only

24. If the final sterile preparation is in a syringe, which of the following statements is TRUE regarding the needle?
    The needle should
    A. remain on the syringe and used for administration
    B. remain on the syringe and replaced just prior to administration
    C. be removed an capped with a sterile tip or cap
    D. be removed and replaced with a clean, unused needle

25. Which of the following is the APPROPRIATE method for removing air bubble from a syringe? 25.____
    A. Pull air into the syringe, shake it vigorously, and depress the plunger
    B. Allow syringe to set for a few minutes, then depress the plunger
    C. Pull plunger back slightly, tap the syringe, and depress the plunger
    D. Pull excess fluid into the syringe, depress plunger to push excess air and fluid into the laminar airflow workbench

KEY (CORRECT ANSWERS)

1.	B	11.	A
2.	C	12.	B
3.	C	13.	A
4.	D	14.	D
5.	C	15.	A
6.	C	16.	B
7.	D	17.	C
8.	A	18.	D
9.	D	19.	A
10.	A	20.	A

21. D
22. A
23. B
24. C
25. B

EXAMINATION SECTION

TEST 1

DIRECTIONS: Each question or incomplete statement is followed by several suggested answers or completions. Select the one that BEST answers the question or completes the statement. *PRINT THE LETTER OF THE CORRECT ANSWER IN THE SPACE AT THE RIGHT.*

1. All of the following are to be included under "Right Documentation" EXCEPT 1.____
   A. name of drug
   B. prescribing physician
   C. route of administration
   D. initial or signature of administering personnel

2. All of the following are goals related to medication safety EXCEPT: 2.____
   A. Improve efficacy of medications
   B. Improve the accuracy of patient identification
   C. Improve effectiveness of communication among caregivers
   D. Reduce risk of health care associated infections

3. All of the following are general guidelines for appropriate drug disposal EXCEPT: 3.____
   A. Follow specific information on the drug label or drug insert
   B. Drug should remain in original container
   C. Unless specifically instructed, do not flush medications down the toilet
   D. Remove drug from original container and dispose in a sealed bag with undesirable substances such as cat litter or coffee grounds

4. All of the following are actions to create safe medication administration EXCEPT: 4.____
   A. Double check all calculated doses
   B. Avoid taking verbal orders
   C. Never use a leading zero (0.5); always use a following zero (5.0)
   D. Avoid easily confused abbreviations

5. The Patient Rights of Medication Safety included all of the following EXCEPT Right 5.____
   A. Drug   B. Dose   C. Time   D. Order

6. Which of the following is NOT a type of medication error? 6.____
   A. Prescribing error   B. Preparation error
   C. Dispensing error   D. Administration error

7. All of the following are considered to be prescribing errors EXCEPT 7.____
   A. patient allergies   B. drug interactions
   C. quantity and refills omitted   D. route not specified

8. Medication Error and Reporting Prevention (MERP) is overseen by which agency?
    A. Institute of Safe Medication Practices
    B. Food and Drug Administration
    C. Institute of Medicine
    D. National Institute of Health

    8.____

9. A telephone order or verbal order for medication must be cosigned by the prescribing health care provider within what time period?
    A. 4 hours   B. 6 hours   C. 12 hours   D. 24 hours

    9.____

10. Which method is incorporated when drugs are stored on the unit and dispensed to all clients from the same container?
    A. Stock drug method   B. Unit dose method
    C. Cart dispensing method   D. Community use method

    10.____

11. Which method is incorporated when drugs are packaged in doses for a 24 hour period by the pharmacy?
    A. Stock drug method   B. Unit dose method
    C. Cart dispensing method   D. Community use method

    11.____

12. Which of the following statements are FALSE regarding the use of the stock drug method?
    A. Drug errors more prevalent
    B. Cost-efficiency of large quantities
    C. Increased opportunity for contamination
    D. Less risk of abuse by health care workers

    12.____

13. Which of the following statements are FALSE regarding the use of the unit dose method?
    A. Immediately replaceable if contaminated
    B. Less chance for contamination and error
    C. Potential delay in receiving the drug
    D. More expensive

    13.____

14. Which agency issues guidelines for the appropriate disposal of prescription drugs?
    A. Institute of Safe Medication Practices
    B. Food and Drug Administration
    C. White House Office of National Drug Control Policy
    D. National Institute of Health

    14.____

15. Which of the following is run by the Food and Drug Administration for reporting serious adverse events, product problems, or medication errors?
    A. MedList   B. MedMark   C. MedWatch   D. MedLink

    15.____

16. Drugs may be administered within what time period before or after the time prescribed?
    A. 15 minutes   B. 30 minutes   C. 60 minutes   D. 120 minutes

17. When the drug has a long half-life, how often is it administered?
    A. Once daily
    B. Twice daily
    C. Once every 48 hours
    D. Several times a day at specific intervals

18. When a drug has a short half-life, how often is it administered?
    A. Once daily
    B. Twice daily
    C. Once every 48 hours
    D. Several times a day at specific intervals

19. Which of the following abbreviations is allowed by the Joint Commission?
    A. U   B. IU   C. b.i.d.   D. q.d.

20. What type of error has occurred if there was a failure to administer an ordered dose to a patient before the next scheduled dose?
    A. Omission error   B. Wrong time error
    C. Unauthorized drug error   D. Improper dose error

21. What type of error has occurred if a patient has been given a dose of a drug that has expired?
    A. Unauthorized drug error   B. Improper dose error
    C. Wrong drug-preparation error   D. Deteriorated drug error

22. Which of the following refers to inappropriate patient behavior regarding adherence to a prescribed medication regimen?
    a. Monitoring error   B. Compliance error
    C. Other medication error   D. Unauthorized drug error

23. Which of the following refers to the failure to review a prescribed regimen for appropriateness and detection of problems?
    A. Monitoring error   B. Compliance error
    C. Other medication error   D. Unauthorized drug error

24. An error that occurred that may have contributed to or directly resulted in death is assigned Category
    A. F   B. G   C. H   D. I

25. If a medication error reaches the patient but did not cause any harm this error is assigned Category
    A. A   B. B   C. C   D. D

KEY (CORRECT ANSWERS)

1.	B	11.	B
2.	A	12.	D
3.	B	13.	A
4.	C	14.	C
5.	D	15.	C
6.	B	16.	C
7.	B	17.	A
8.	A	18.	D
9.	D	19.	C
10.	A	20.	A

21. D
22. B
23. A
24. D
25. C

TEST 2

DIRECTIONS: Each question or incomplete statement is followed by several suggested answers or completions. Select the one that BEST answers the question or completes the statement. *PRINT THE LETTER OF THE CORRECT ANSWER IN THE SPACE AT THE RIGHT.*

1. How many times should a medication be checked prior to administration? 1.____
   A. 1   B. 2   C. 3   D. 4

2. A "Stat" order should be administered within what period of time? 2.____
   A. 5 minutes   B. 10 minutes   C. 15 minutes   D. 20 minutes

3. A "Now" order must be administered within what period of time? 3.____
   A. 3-5 minutes   B. 10-15 minutes
   C. 20-30 minutes   D. 30-90 minutes

4. Needleless syringes should be used to measure amounts under what volume? 4.____
   A. 3 ml   B. 5 ml   C. 10 ml   D. 20 ml

5. Reconstituted solutions must be used within what time period? 5.____
   A. 24 hours   B. 7 days   C. 14 days   D. 21 days

6. A transdermal patch should be labeled with all of the following EXCEPT 6.____
   A. date   B. time applied
   C. initials   D. time to be removed

7. A patient should be instructed to hold their breath for _____ seconds after inhaling medication. 7.____
   A. 5   B. 10   C. 20   D. 30

8. If a spacer is used in conjunction with an inhaled medication, what percentage more medication is deposited in the lungs? 8.____
   A. 50%   B. 60%   C. 70%   D. 80%

9. A patient should be instructed to rinse their mouth following the administration of any inhalant containing a corticosteroid due to risk of ____ infection. 9.____
   A. fungal   B. bacterial   C. viral   D. prion

10. The ISMP, FDA, and Joint Commission have promoted the use of which of the following to reduce confusion between similar drug names? 10.____
    A. Abbreviations   B. Generic names
    C. Trade names   D. Tallman letters

11. All of the following units have a high incidence of preventable medication errors EXCEPT
    A. operating room
    B. emergency room
    C. pediatric units
    D. intensive care units

12. HEPA filters remove 99.97% of air particles of what size or larger?
    A. 0.05mm   B. 0.1mm   C. 0.2mm   D. 0.3mm

13. Airborne precautions are recommended for a patient with all of the following medical conditions EXCEPT
    A. MRSA
    B. tuberculosis
    C. measles
    D. chickenpox

14. Contact precautions are recommended for patients with which of the following medical conditions?
    A. VRE
    B. Tuberculosis
    C. Measles
    D. Chickenpox

15. What piece of legislation authorized the creation of Patient Safety Organizations to improve quality and safety of the health care delivery in the United States?
    A. Affordable Care Act
    B. Patient Safety and Quality Improvement Act
    C. Emergency Medical Treatment and Active Labor Act
    D. Health Insurance Portability and Accountability Act

16. Which federal agency provides provisions for the Patient Safety and Quality Improvement Act?
    A. Food and Drug Administration
    B. Centers for Disease Control and Prevention
    C. Agency for Healthcare Research and Quality
    D. World Health Organization

17. Which of the following is a proactive tool to prevent medication errors?
    A. Root Cause Analysis
    B. Failure Mode Effects Analysis
    C. Mixed Methods Analysis
    D. Analysis of Mortalities

18. Which of the following is a retrospective investigation of an event that has already occurred?
    A. Root cause analysis
    B. Failure mode effects analysis
    C. Mixed methods analysis
    D. Analysis of Mortalities

19. Which abbreviation should be used for micrograms?
    A. mg   B. µ   C. mcg   D. µcg

20. Which medication should be spelled out instead of using MS or MSO$_4$ abbreviations?
    A. Magnesium Sulfate
    B. Morphine Sulfate
    C. Manganese Sulfate
    D. Mercury Sulfate

21. What color script pad should controlled drugs be written on?
    A. Normal white
    B. Special pink
    C. Special blue
    D. Special green

22. Which of the following is a safety program to minimize risks while preserving the benefit of the product which is required by 225 medications?
    A. Risk Evaluation and Mitigation Strategy
    B. Vaccine Adverse Event Reporting System
    C. Manufacturer and user facility device experience database
    D. Failure Mode Effects Analysis

23. Which of the following is defined as a lack of treatment intensification or therapy underuse which may contribute to 80% of all heart attacks and strokes?
    A. Sentinel Event
    B. Clinical Error
    C. Clinical Inertia
    D. Polypharmacy

24. Prescribing errors are inappropriately selecting a drug based on all of the following EXCEPT
    A. contraindications
    B. known allergies
    C. existing drug therapies
    D. efficacy of the drug

25. What phenomenon is defined as the process whereby side effects of drugs are misdiagnosed as symptoms of another medical condition in which further medications are administered to treat?
    A. Clinical Inertia
    B. Polypharmacy
    C. Prescribing Cascade
    D. Medication Error

KEY (CORRECT ANSWERS)

1. C
2. C
3. D
4. C
5. C

6. D
7. B
8. D
9. A
10. D

11. A
12. D
13. A
14. A
15. B

16. C
17. B
18. A
19. C
20. B

21. C
22. A
23. C
24. D
25. C

EXAMINATION SECTION

TEST 1

DIRECTIONS: Each question or incomplete statement is followed by several suggested answers or completions. Select the one that BEST answers the question or completes the statement. *PRINT THE LETTER OF THE CORRECT ANSWER IN THE SPACE AT THE RIGHT.*

1. All of the following statements are true regarding quality assurance EXCEPT: 1.____
   A. Uses total quality management
   B. Monitored through audits
   C. Guided by standard operating procedures
   D. Ensures quality of product by using quality procedures

2. All of the following statements are true regarding quality control EXCEPT: 2.____
   A. Follows standard operating procedures to assure quality, purity, and effectiveness
   B. Uses total quality management
   C. Monitored through audits
   D. Daily control of quality

3. Facilities that are performing sterile compounding must adhere to USP _____ requirements. 3.____
   A. 794   B. 795   C. 796   D. 797

4. Facilities that are performing non-sterile compounding must adhere to USP _____ requirements. 4.____
   A. 794   B. 795   C. 796   D. 797

5. Which organization established the "Do Not Use List"? 5.____
   A. Institution for Safe Medical Practices
   B. Joint Commission
   C. Food and Drug Administration
   D. United States Pharmacopeia

6. Which organization established the "Do Not Crush List"? 6.____
   A. Institution for Safe Medical Practices
   B. Joint Commission
   C. Food and Drug Administration
   D. United States Pharmacopeia

7. What type of drug recall results in permanent harm or death to a patient? 7.____
   A. Class I   B. Class II   C. Class III   D. Class IV

8. Which organization establishes the standards for medications?
    A. Institution for Safe Medical Practices
    B. Joint Commission
    C. Food and Drug Administration
    D. United States Pharmacopeia

    8.____

9. Which of the following is a function of the United States Pharmacopeia?
    A. Sets standards for ID, strength, quality, and purity
    B. Oversees food, drugs, medical devices, cosmetics, and tobacco
    C. Accredits and certifies health care organizations
    D. Approves vet drugs and adverse events

    9.____

10. Which of the following is a function of the Food and Drug Administration?
    A. Limit adulterants in dietary supplements
    B. Oversees allergenics, vaccines, blood, shortages, and recalls
    C. Sets safety goals and protocols for certified facilities
    D. Certification for disease care and home care

    10.____

11. Which of the following is a function of the Joint Commission?
    A. Approves all devices, implants, diagnostic, recalls, and alerts
    B. Issues warning letters for specific meds and watches new meds
    C. Accredits and certifies health care organizations
    D. Issues black box warnings

    11.____

12. Which of the following is a function of the Institution for Safe Medical Practices?
    A. Addresses infections and patient safety concerns
    B. Issues error prone abbreviations list
    C. Evaluates radiation
    D. Develops policies on biotechnology and dietary supplements

    12.____

13. All of the following are reportable to the Institution for Safe Medical Practices-Medication Error Report Program EXCEPT
    A. errors in prescribing, transcribing, dispensing, and monitoring
    B. look-alike sound-like drugs or similar packaging
    C. vaccine errors
    D. wrong route

    13.____

14. All of the following are reportable to the Institution for Safe Medical Practices-Vaccine Adverse Effect Reporting System EXCEPT
    A. wrong drug, strength, dose
    B. misuse of medical devices
    C. calculation or prep area
    D. medications error

    14.____

15. Which organization developed the Pharmacy Tech Initiative?
    A. American Pharmacists Association
    B. American Society of Health System Pharmacists
    C. Accrediting Council of Pharmacy Education
    D. State Boards of Pharmacy

15.____

16. Which organization is a valuable resource for information and education for both pharmacists and pharmacy technicians?
    A. American Pharmacists Association
    B. American Society of Health System Pharmacists
    C. Accrediting Council of Pharmacy Education
    D. State Boards of Pharmacy

16.____

17. Which organization ensures quality by setting standards in education and continuing education?
    A. National Association of Boards of Pharmacy
    B. American Society of Health System Pharmacists
    C. Accrediting Council of Pharmacy Education
    D. State Boards of Pharmacy

17.____

18. Disciplining pharmacies and pharmacy employees is the responsibility of which organization?
    A. Joint Commission
    B. Food and Drug Administration
    C. Accrediting Council of Pharmacy Education
    D. State Boards of Pharmacy

18.____

19. Which organization is responsible for assisting State Boards of Pharmacy regarding standards for public health?
    A. National Association of Boards of Pharmacy
    B. American Society of Health System Pharmacists
    C. Accrediting Council of Pharmacy Education
    D. State Boards of Pharmacy

19.____

20. The _____ is responsible for safety data sheets maintained in pharmacies.
    A. State Boards of Pharmacy
    B. National Association of Boards in Pharmacy
    C. Occupational Safety and Health Administration
    D. American Pharmacists Association

20.____

21. _____ are written rules of an organization that must be followed.
    A. Policies   B. Procedures   C. Guidelines   D. Standards

21.____

22. _____ are processes employees must follow during each task to ensure consistency.
    A. Policies   B. Procedures   C. Guidelines   D. Standards

22.____

23. All of the following statements are true regarding pharmacists EXCEPT:
    A. They graduate from an accredited school of pharmacy with a B.S. in Pharmacy or a PharmD.
    B. They maintain 20 hours of continuing education every two years with one year regarding law.
    C. Their licenses can go to other states without taking exam but might need to take law exam.
    D. They must meet state requirements for license, exam, and continuing education.

23.____

24. All of the following are true regarding pharmacy technicians EXCEPT:
    A. They need a high school diploma or GED.
    B. They graduate from an accredited school of pharmacy with a B.S. in Pharmacy.
    C. They maintain 20 hours of continuing education every two years with one year regarding law.
    D. Some states require registration with the Board of Pharmacy.

24.____

25. All of the following statements are true regarding hospital automatic processing of med orders EXCEPT:
    A. Order entered into hospital computer that gives order to the pharmacy
    B. Ordering physician reviews and verifies the order
    C. RN retrieves the medication from point-of-use med station
    D. Pharmacy technician fills inventory as med supply falls below periodic automatic replacement levels

25.____

KEY (CORRECT ANSWERS)

1. A
2. C
3. D
4. C
5. B

6. A
7. A
8. D
9. A
10. B

11. C
12. B
13. C
14. D
15. B

16. A
17. C
18. D
19. A
20. C

21. A
22. B
23. B
24. B
25. B

TEST 2

DIRECTIONS: Each question or incomplete statement is followed by several suggested answers or completions. Select the one that BEST answers the question or completes the statement. *PRINT THE LETTER OF THE CORRECT ANSWER IN THE SPACE AT THE RIGHT.*

1. Which guidelines for the quality assurance of products, according to the American Society of Health System Pharmacists, include products compounded from non-sterile parts before sterilized or prepared with sterile or non-sterile ingredients with open system transfer prior to sterilization? 1.____
   A. Level 1　　　B. Level 2　　　C. Level 3　　　D. Level 4

2. Which guidelines for the quality assurance of products, according to the American Society of Health System Pharmacists, include products stored at room temperature and administered within 28 hours of preparation, products prepared for more than one person, and prepared by aseptic transfer of non-pyrogenic sterile products? 2.____
   A. Level 1　　　B. Level 2　　　C. Level 3　　　D. Level 4

3. Which guidelines for the quality assurance of products, according to the American Society of Health System Pharmacists, include products stored at room temperature and administered more than 28 hours after preparation, products batch prepared with no preservatives for more than one person, TPN like compounding of sterile ingredients using close system aseptic transfer? 3.____
   A. Level 1　　　B. Level 2　　　C. Level 3　　　D. Level 4

4. Which of the following informs the pharmacist of any drug interactions or contraindications a patient can be susceptible to while taking a medication? 4.____
   A. ISMP-MERP　　　　　　　　B. ISMP-VAERS
   C. Drug Utilization Evaluation　　D. Drug Reconciliation

5. Which of the following is the process of verifying with patients the medications they are currently taking? 5.____
   A. ISMP-MERP　　　　　　　　B. ISMP-VAERS
   C. Drug Utilization Evaluation　　D. Drug Reconciliation

6. All of the following statements are true regarding quality assurance for medication distribution EXCEPT: 6.____
   A. Bar-coded labels should be used to streamline the process and reduce error
   B. Automation should be used to track and regulate substances
   C. Robotics can be used to scan unit dose medications
   D. Floor stock inventory is preferred to unit dose systems in the hospital environment

7. All of the following are beneficial for preventing medication errors EXCEPT:
   A. NDC number from prescription label must match bulk med label
   B. Prescription and medication orders should be reviewed two times
   C. Prescription label should be compared with original prescription to ensure accuracy
   D. Pharmacies required to have a library relevant to the practice of pharmacy

8. _____ is a good practice to perform prior to dispensing narcotics and after the narcotics order has been verified by a pharmacist or pharmacy technician.
   A. Reconciling
   B. Justifying
   C. Double counting
   D. Restocking

9. All of the following statements are true regarding MedWatch EXCEPT:
   A. FDA's safety info and adverse event reporting program
   B. Has online voluntary report form to report adverse events with drugs, devices, products, and cosmetics
   C. Is also used to report vaccines
   D. Provides safety alerts

10. All of the following statements are true regarding the FDS adverse event reporting system (FAERS) EXCEPT:
    A. Database on adverse events and med error reports given to the FDA
    B. Collects data from adverse events after vaccines and reports safety concerns
    C. Information used to identify possible safety concerns
    D. Manufacturers who receive adverse drug event report must submit info to the FDA

11. All of the following statements are true regarding FDA product recalls EXCEPT:
    A. Pharmacy is notified by the FDA, manufacturer, or wholesaler by mail or fax
    B. Pharmacy contacts patients with recalled product and it should be returned for refund or substitution
    C. Recalled medication returned to the FDA for credit
    D. Pharmacy technician should reorder the medication, notify physician, and ask if the ordered medical should be changed

12. A _____ permits the nursing staff to verify controlled substances at each change of shift by monitoring receipt, administration, and disposal.
    A. Controlled Substance Form
    B. Medical Administration Record
    C. Medication Delivery Record
    D. Physician Order Sheet

13. Which of the following documents medications administered to a patient with drug, dose, route, frequency, times, allergies, and diagnoses?
    A. Controlled Substance Form
    B. Medical Administration Record
    C. Medication Delivery Record
    D. Physician Order Sheet

14. A _____ includes non-drug orders such as diets, allergies, therapies, and diagnoses.
    A. Controlled Substance Form
    B. Medical Administration Record
    C. Medication Delivery Record
    D. Physician Order Sheet

15. Which of the following documents external treatments given to patients in the hospital or long-term care facilities?
    A. Medication Administration Record
    B. Physician Order Sheet
    C. Resident Monitoring Form
    D. Treatment Administration Record

16. A _____ documents behavior of patients and other factors such as intervention, outcomes, and adverse reactions.
    A. Medication Administration Record
    B. Physician Order Sheet
    C. Resident Monitoring Form
    D. Treatment Administration Record

17. All of the following statements are true regarding working conditions in a pharmacy EXCEPT:
    A. There is a maximum number of prescriptions a pharmacist may fill during a shift.
    B. The State Board of Pharmacy limits the number of hours worked in a given pay period.
    C. A pharmacist can supervise a maximum of four pharmacy technicians during a shift.
    D. The State Board of Pharmacy requires a pharmacist to take at least four vacation days every three months.

18. Which of the following is defined as bringing people together with different expertise to work on the same task for improved lateral communication for better problem solving?
    A. Cross Training
    B. Multi-skilling
    C. Multi-tasking
    D. Job Sharing

19. _____ is defined as team members trained in skills to perform more than one job.
    A. Cross Training
    B. Multi-skilling
    C. Multi-tasking
    D. Job Sharing

20. All of the following are characteristics associated with efficiency EXCEPT
    A. inventory turnover rates
    B. absenteeism and tardiness through payroll
    C. reduction in prescription errors per shift
    D. average wait time per prescription

21. Which of the following is a characteristic associated with productivity?
    A. Prescriptions filled per hour
    B. Compliance reports from vendors
    C. Reduction in prescription errors per shift
    D. Inventory turnover rates

22. _____ is defined as a philosophy of continual improvement for the process associated with providing a good or service that meets or exceeds customer expectation.
    A. Customer service
    B. Continuous quality improvement
    C. Quality assurance
    D. Quality control

23. All of the following are other names for continuous quality improvement EXCEPT
    A. Quality Process Management
    B. Quality Improvement Process
    C. Total Quality Management
    D. Total Quality Control

24. All of the following are legal reasons for pharmacy quality commitment EXCEPT
    A. Federal legislation
    B. Medicare
    C. third party contracts
    D. lower insurance rates

25. All of the following are characteristics of a sentinel system EXCEPT
    A. problems and errors become more frequent
    B. assembly line-like
    C. reduces confusion
    D. standardized workflow process of filling a prescription

KEY (CORRECT ANSWERS)

1. C
2. A
3. B
4. C
5. D

6. D
7. B
8. C
9. C
10. B

11. C
12. A
13. B
14. D
15. D

16. C
17. D
18. A
19. B
20. B

21. A
22. B
23. A
24. D
25. A

EXAMINATION SECTION
TEST 1

DIRECTIONS: Each question or incomplete statement is followed by several suggested answers or completions. Select the one that BEST answers the question or completes the statement. *PRINT THE LETTER OF THE CORRECT ANSWER IN THE SPACE AT THE RIGHT.*

1. Which of the following statements is true regarding measurement of a liquid in a graduated cylinder?   1.____
   A. Liquids are measured at eye level by reading the bottom of the meniscus.
   B. Liquids are measured at eye level by reading the top of the meniscus.
   C. Liquids that form an upside down meniscus are measured at eye level by reading the midpoint between the top and bottom of the meniscus.
   D. Liquids that form an upside down meniscus are measured at eye level by reading the lowest point.

2. The part of the prescription that provides directions to the patient such as "avoid sunlight" is referred to as   2.____
   A. subscription   B. inscription
   C. superscription   D. signa

3. The part of the prescription that includes the name and strength of the medication prescribed and the amount prescribed is referred to as   3.____
   A. subscription   B. inscription
   C. superscription   D. signa

4. The _____ is the part of the subscription that includes directions to the pharmacist for dispensing the medication.   4.____
   A. subscription   B. inscription
   C. superscription   D. signa

5. All of the following are included in a superscription EXCEPT   5.____
   A. patient's name   B. directions for the patient
   C. Rx symbol   D. date the prescription was written

6. Which of the following is a type of medication order that is written by a physician if a patient is being admitted to a hospital?   6.____
   A. Stat order   B. Discharge order
   C. Admission order   D. PRN order

7. All of the following should be included on an admission order EXCEPT   7.____
   A. drugs the patient is currently taking
   B. weight and height of the patient
   C. any allergies
   D. medications the patient has previously taken

8. A _____ order is a type of medication order sent to the pharmacy that must be filled immediately.
   A. PRN   B. Stat   C. Now   D. admission

9. Which type of medication order is given on an as needed basis for specific signs and symptoms exhibited by the patient?
   A. Stat   B. Discharge   C. Admission   D. PRN

10. Which of the following is a drug used in a hospital or other inpatient setting that is prepackaged from bulk for a single administration for one patient?
    A. Bulk dose
    B. Unit dose
    C. Lot dose
    D. Packaged dose

11. All of the following are parts of a written prescription EXCEPT
    A. inscription
    B. transcription
    C. subscription
    D. superscription

12. _____ is part of a prescription that when checked indicates the generic drug must not be dispensed and brand name is required.
    A. No substitutions
    B. Brand name only
    C. Dispense as written
    D. No generics

13. Which of the following is a bright, colorful label placed on the bottle to provide information in addition to what is on the bottle label such as alerts to patients for specific information to which careful attention is to be paid?
    A. Container label
    B. Warning label
    C. Auxiliary label
    D. Precautionary label

14. All of the following should be placed on the prescription container level EXCEPT
    A. directions for use
    B. initials of dispensing pharmacist
    C. patient diagnosis
    D. prescription Rx number

15. A spatula is used to count in what quantities?
    A. 1   B. 5   C. 10   D. 20

16. All of the following are tasks performed by pharmacy technicians EXCEPT
    A. interpret prescription signa
    B. count and pour correct medication
    C. administer unit doses
    D. bill prescription to third part prescription providers

17. If a prescription is coded DAW 2, which of the following does this code suggest?
    Substitution allowed,
    A. patient requested product dispensed
    B. pharmacist selected product dispensed
    C. generic drug not in stock
    D. brand drug dispensed as generic

18. If a drug cannot be substituted and the brand name drug is mandated by law, what code should accompany the prescription?
    A. DAW 4
    B. DAW 5
    C. DAW 6
    D. DAW 7

19. If a drug is able to be substituted because the generic drug is not available in the marketplace, what code should accompany this prescription?
    A. DAW 6
    B. DAW 7
    C. DAW 8
    D. DAW 9

20. Which of the following would be an appropriate auxiliary label for a suspension?
    A. Apply to skin
    B. For external use only
    C. Avoid sunlight
    D. Shake well

21. Which of the following would be an appropriate auxiliary label for a transdermal patch?
    A. Apply to skin
    B. For external use only
    C. For topical use only
    D. Avoid bathing

22. What type of dosing system combines unit dose medications that are blister-packed onto a card instead of a box?
    A. Unit dose
    B. Modified unit dose
    C. Blended unit dose
    D. Childproof unit dose

23. All of the following medications would be dispensed from a dropper bottle EXCEPT
    A. ophthalmic liquids
    B. oral liquids
    C. liquids used for wound or skin care
    D. otic liquids

24. What type of container is impervious to air or gas?
    A. Light resistant
    B. Hermetic
    C. Tight
    D. Well-closed

25. What type of container is designed to hold a quantity of drug product for administration as a single dose?
    A. Single unit
    B. Single dose
    C. Unit dose
    D. Unit of use

KEY (CORRECT ANSWERS)

1.	A	11.	B
2.	D	12.	C
3.	B	13.	C
4.	A	14.	C
5.	B	15.	B
6.	C	16.	C
7.	D	17.	A
8.	B	18.	D
9.	D	19.	C
10.	B	20.	D

21. A
22. B
23. C
24. B
25. A

TEST 2

DIRECTIONS: Each question or incomplete statement is followed by several suggested answers or completions. Select the one that BEST answers the question or completes the statement. *PRINT THE LETTER OF THE CORRECT ANSWER IN THE SPACE AT THE RIGHT.*

1. What is meant by the abbreviation "hs"? 1.____
   A. Morning   B. Hour   C. At bedtime   D. As needed

2. What is meant by the abbreviation "au"? 2.____
   A. As soon as possible   B. Each ear
   C. Each eye   D. Before meals

3. What is meant by the abbreviation "gtt"? 3.____
   A. Oral   B. Topical   C. Drops   D. Injection

4. What is meant by the abbreviation "pc"? 4.____
   A. Before meals   B. After meals
   C. As needed   D. Nothing by mouth

5. What is meant by the abbreviation "os"? 5.____
   A. Both eyes   B. Right eye
   C. Left eye   D. Both ears

6. What abbreviation would be used if a medication is supposed to be given every other day? 6.____
   A. qd   B. qod   C. qid   D. bid

7. Which medication should be dispensed in the original manufacturer's bottle? 7.____
   A. Digoxin   B. Coumadin   C. Insulin   D. Nitrostat

8. What do the middle four numbers of an NDC number represent? 8.____
   A. Drug manufacturer   B. Drug entity
   C. Drug package   D. Drug expiration date

9. What is the FIRST step in the medication fill process? 9.____
   A. Enter prescription information into the computer
   B. Obtain a prescription label and compare it to the original prescription to check accuracy
   C. Obtain prescription from patient
   D. Pull appropriate medication from the shelf using the NDC number to confirm the correct medication was selected

10. A monthly pack of birth control pills or a four-pack of medication taken once a week for a month is an example of a ____ container. 10.____
    A. Single unit   B. Single dose
    C. Unit dose`   D. Unit of use

11. What type of container is used for bulk powders or large quantities of tablets, capsules, and viscous liquid?
    A. Round vials
    B. Wide mouth bottles
    C. Dropper bottles
    D. Applicator bottles

    11.____

12. Collapsible tubes are used to dispense which of the following?
    A. Suppositories
    B. Powders
    C. Semisolids
    D. Liquids

    12.____

13. Which of the following is a disadvantage for a centralized pharmacy?
    A. Bar code scanning for accurate med dispensing
    B. Inability to handle all dosage forms
    C. Eliminates or reduces management issues
    D. Active alerts for safety for high risk medications

    13.____

14. All of the following are characteristics of the Pyxis MedStation System EXCEPT
    A. Bar code scanning for accurate med dispensing
    B. Active alerts for safety for high risk meds
    C. Prevent loading of wrong medication
    D. Tracks and monitors replenishment of controlled substance inventory in a hospital

    14.____

15. What dispensing system restricts access to only one medication at a time to reduce risk?
    A. Pyxis MedStation System
    B. Cubie System
    C. Pyxis CII Safe
    D. Pyxis Anesthesia System

    15.____

16. What dispensing system tracks and monitors replenishment of controlled substance inventory in a hospital?
    A. Pyxis MedStation System
    B. Cubie System
    C. Pyxis CII Safe
    D. Pyxis Anesthesia System

    16.____

17. What dispensing system offers a variety of drawer types and a controlled access drawer for high-risk medications?
    A. Pyxis MedStation System
    B. Cubie System
    C. Pyxis CII Safe
    D. Pyxis Anesthesia System

    17.____

18. A prescription is written for 2gtt AU BID. The label placed on the patient's medication reads two drops in
    A. the left eye two times daily
    B. the right ear three times a day
    C. both ears two times daily
    D. both eyes two times daily

    18.____

19. What information is required on the medication label of a prepackaged or repackaged unit dose medication in an inpatient setting?
    A. Patient's name, date of birth, name of medication, and direction of use
    B. Medication name and strength, lot number, and expiration date
    C. Medication name and strength, lot number, and directions for use
    D. Patient's name, pharmacy name and address, physician's name, and number of refills

20. Which of the following would be an appropriate auxiliary label placed on containers of anti-infective agents?
    A. Take with dairy products
    B. Avoid dairy products
    C. May cause drowsiness
    D. Finish all this medication unless otherwise directed by the prescriber

21. How many capsules would be in a 30-day prescription to be administered qd?
    A. 15   B. 30   C. 60   D. 90

22. Prescribers must use tamper-resistant prescriptions for which group of patients?
    A. Children   B. Elderly
    C. Medicare patients   D. Medicaid patients

23. What type of order states a patient receives a specific medication at a specific time each day while in the hospital?
    A. Standing order   B. Admission order
    C. PRN order   D. STAT order

24. How many teaspoon doses are in one pint of elixir?
    A. 12   B. 24   C. 48   D. 96

25. How many milligrams (mg) are there in one grain (gr)?
    A. 45   B. 55   C. 65   D. 75

KEY (CORRECT ANSWERS)

1.	C	11.	B
2.	B	12.	C
3.	C	13.	B
4.	B	14.	D
5.	C	15.	B
6.	B	16.	C
7.	D	17.	D
8.	B	18.	C
9.	C	19.	B
10.	D	20.	D

21. B
22. D
23. A
24. D
25. C

EXAMINATION SECTION

TEST 1

DIRECTIONS: Each question or incomplete statement is followed by several suggested answers or completions. Select the one that BEST answers the question or completes the statement. *PRINT THE LETTER OF THE CORRECT ANSWER IN THE SPACE AT THE RIGHT.*

1. Which of the following is an inventory of all controlled substances prior to opening a new pharmacy or when there is a change of pharmacist in charge?
    A. Initial inventory
    B. Biennial inventory
    C. Perpetual inventory
    D. Physical inventory

    1.____

2. A(n) _____ inventory reflects exactly what is on hand at a particular time and is often maintained on Class II medications.
    A. initial
    B. biennial
    C. perpetual
    D. physical

    2.____

3. Which of the following is a type of inventory required by the DEA of all controlled substances every two years in which Class II medications must be accurately counted and Class III, IV, and V medications can be estimated?
    A. Initial inventory
    B. Biennial inventory
    C. Perpetual inventory
    D. Physical inventory

    3.____

4. A(n) _____ inventory is performed on an annual basis to determine what is on hand at a particular time and the value of inventory is based on the cost of the items.
    A. initial
    B. biennial
    C. perpetual
    D. physical

    4.____

5. Which of the following is an inventory auditing procedure in which a small subset of inventory is counted on a specific day?
    A. Basic count
    B. Stock count
    C. Cycle count
    D. Perpetual count

    5.____

6. The _____ is a cycle count method which emphasized inventory value with items of a higher determined value being counted more often and items with a lower value counted less frequently.
    A. Pareto Method
    B. Hybrid Cycle Counting Methods
    C. Cycle Counting by Usage
    D. Economic Approach

    6.____

7. The Pareto Method is commonly referred to as the _____ Rule.
    A. 50-50
    B. 60-40
    C. 70-30
    D. 80-20

    7.____

8. All of the following are considered to be advantages of cycle counting EXCEPT:
    A. Improves the gross margin return on investment
    B. Allows for overstocking of frequently used items
    C. Establishes a true just-in-time inventory count
    D. Efficiently controls inventories of expensive items

    8.____

9. All of the following are considered to be disadvantages of cycle counting EXCEPT:
   A. Identifies slow-moving items
   B. Inconsistency contributes to errors
   C. Can be disruptive to business operations
   D. Lag times between the count and entering the inventory into the data management system contributes to variances in inventory counts

9._____

10. Most hospital pharmacies have medications organized according to a precise system. Initially, medications are categorized and organized based on which of the following?
    A. Drug classification
    B. Specific route of administration
    C. Generic name
    D. Brand name

10._____

11. Once medications are initially categorized and organized, what is the next criteria for organization?
    A. Alphabetically according to generic name
    B. Alphabetically according to brand name
    C. According to drug classification
    D. Numerically according to NDC number

11._____

12. According to manufacturer's instructions, where should most vaccines be stored?
    A. Negative pressure room
    B. In the refrigerator
    C. In a secure area of the pharmacy separate from other medications
    D. In original packaging

12._____

13. _____ are usually stored in a secure area of the pharmacy, separate from other medications.
    A. Narcotics
    B. Vaccines
    C. Anti-psychotics
    D. Antibiotics

13._____

14. What is the appropriate time frame for holding a product prior to returning it to stock?
    A. 24-72 hours   B. 3-5 days   C. 5-7 days   D. 7-10 days

14._____

15. Which of the following occurs when a product has a minor violation that would not be subject to FDA legal action?
    A. Class I Recall
    B. Class II Recall
    C. Class III Recall
    D. Market Withdrawal

15._____

16. For what time period should brand name products be managed down prior to the introduction of a generic drug into the market?
    A. 30-60 days   B. 60-90 days   C. 90-120 days   D. 120-180 days

16._____

17. Product recalls and brand-to-generic transitions decrease the dollar value of inventory. This reduction is referred to as
    A. Negative Inventory Event
    B. Positive Inventory Event
    C. Price Restructuring
    D. Inventory Adjustment

    17._____

18. Return-to-stock items and the receipt of new products increase the dollar value of the inventory. This increase is referred to as
    A. Negative Inventory Event
    B. Positive Inventory Event
    C. Price Restructuring
    D. Inventory Adjustment

    18._____

19. Under what circumstances would a product recall positively impact the inventory of a pharmacy?
    Recalled product
    A. substituted with a less expensive product
    B. substituted with a more expensive product
    C. not issued a substitute
    D. is reinstated

    19._____

20. Recent legislation has placed limitations on the dispensing of medications in which of the following?
    A. Hospitals
    B. Physician Offices
    C. Outpatient Clinics
    D. Long-term Care Facilities

    20._____

21. New legislation has limited pharmacies in long-term care facilities to dispensing no more than a _____ day supply of medication.
    A. 3   B. 5   C. 7-14   D. 30

    21._____

22. _____ measures the operational costs and profitability of a pharmacy.
    A. Gross Margin Return on Investment
    B. Carrying Costs
    C. Procurement Costs
    D. Inventory Turns

    22._____

23. Which of the following refers to the number of times per year inventory is sold and replaced at cost?
    A. Cycle Counting
    B. Inventory Turns
    C. Procurement Costs
    D. Carrying Costs

    23._____

24. _____ are all costs associated with maintaining inventories.
    A. Operating costs
    B. Inventory turns
    C. Procurement costs
    D. Carrying costs

    24._____

25. _____ Stock is the amount of inventory carried to account for fluctuations in demand and in order cycle times.
    A. Basic   B. Back   C. Safety   D. Over

    25._____

KEY (CORRECT ANSWERS)

1.	A	11.	A
2.	C	12.	B
3.	B	13.	A
4.	D	14.	D
5.	C	15.	D
6.	A	16.	A
7.	D	17.	A
8.	B	18.	B
9.	A	19.	B
10.	B	20.	D

21. C
22. A
23. B
24. D
25. C

TEST 2

DIRECTIONS: Each question or incomplete statement is followed by several suggested answers or completions. Select the one that BEST answers the question or completes the statement. *PRINT THE LETTER OF THE CORRECT ANSWER IN THE SPACE AT THE RIGHT.*

1. The Omnibus Reconciliation Act of 1990 mandated the pharmacist provide which of the following with each prescription dispensed and increased the need for a pharmacy technician to assist in product dispensing?
    A. Treatment Alternatives
    B. Patient Counseling
    C. MSDS Sheets
    D. Possible Drug Interactions

    1.____

2. _____ formulary carries all pharmaceutical products using multiple tiered pricing with a distinct price for branded, generic, lifestyle, and drugs not covered?
    A. Open   B. Closed   C. Restricted   D. Exclusive

    2.____

3. A(n) _____ Formulary offers a limited number of products of each covered drug classification.
    A. Open   B. Closed   C. Restricted   D. Exclusive

    3.____

4. A(n) _____ Formulary is a selective, limited, and partially closed formulary when some non-formulary medications.
    A. Open   B. Closed   C. Restricted   D. Exclusive

    4.____

5. All of the following are classified as hazardous waste EXCEPT
    A. drugs with more than one active ingredient
    B. Chemotherapeutic agents
    C. Drugs with LD50's
    D. Endocrine disruptors

    5.____

6. Which of the following is a detailed summary of purchasing history based on the 80/20 rule, designating medications that account for 80% of the drugs costs for that period of time?
    A. Compliance Report
    B. Inventory Summary
    C. Velocity Report
    D. Utilization Review

    6.____

7. At what temperature should the freezer in the pharmacy be maintained?
    A. -10 to 0°C   B. -15 to -5°C   C. -25 to -10°C   D. -30 to -15°C

    7.____

8. If medications are to be stored in a "dry temperature," humidity cannot exceed what percentage at controlled room temperature?
    A. 20%   B. 30%   C. 40%   D. 50%

    8.____

9. _____ is defined as the rate in which inventory is used, generally expressed in number of days.
    A. Usage
    B. Administration
    C. Cycle Counting
    D. Turnover

    9.____

10. Which of the following is a drug product that when administered in the same amount will provide the same therapeutic effect and pharmacokinetic characteristics as another drug with which it is compared?
    A. Treatment equivalent
    B. Treatment substitution
    C. Therapeutic equivalent
    D. Therapeutic substitution

    10.____

11. What is the purpose of a group purchasing organization for a hospital pharmacy?
    A. Negotiate prices with drug manufacturers
    B. Negotiate prices with a local drug wholesaler
    C. Purchase drugs from a drug manufacturer for the hospital
    D. Purchase drugs from a local drug wholesaler

    11.____

12. Which of the following is a substitution of one medication for another medication that is not generically equivalent but has the same therapeutic effect?
    A. Treatment equivalent
    B. Therapeutic interchange
    C. Therapeutic equivalent
    D. Therapeutic substitution

    12.____

13. Which of the following is a list of items that are in short supply and need to be ordered or reordered from a vendor?
    A. Closed Formulary
    B. Restricted Formulary
    C. Want List
    D. Short List

    13.____

14. _____ Vendor Agreement is an agreement between a pharmacy and a wholesaler in which the pharmacy agrees to purchase the majority of its products from that wholesaler in return for other consideration?
    A. Prime   B. Exclusive   C. Restricted   D. Closed

    14.____

15. A(n) _____ is a method to identify and define inventory items based on their usage in which products are ranked based on their purchase history and dollar amount of total annual costs and is focused on the products that will have the greatest inventory turnover rate.
    A. Compliance Report
    B. Utilization Review
    C. ABC Analysis
    D. Velocity Report

    15.____

16. All of the following are included as members of the Pharmacy and Therapeutics Committee who develop a formulary for a hospital EXCEPT
    A. pharmacists
    B. pharmacy technicians
    C. physicians
    D. nurses

    16.____

17. When performing an ABC analysis, "A" items represent _____ of inventory and _____ of total sales.
    A. 20%; 70%   B. 30%; 20%   C. 50%; 10%   D. 70%; 30%

    17.____

18. When performing an ABC analysis, "B" items represent _____ of inventory and _____ of total sales.
    A. 20%; 70%   B. 30%; 20%   C. 50%; 10%   D. 70%; 30%

    18.____

19. When performing an ABC analysis, "C" items represent _____ of inventory and _____ of total sales.
    A. 20%; 70%   B. 30%; 20%   C. 50%; 10%   D. 70%; 30%

20. Which of the following is direct transmission of prescriptions from physicians to the pharmacy which helps minimize errors due to illegibility in handwriting and helps to reduce the potential for forged prescriptions from drug-seeking patients?
    A. Computer-Physician Order Entry
    B. Electronic Medication Administration Record
    C. E-Prescribing
    D. Direct Entry

21. _____ is electronic documentation of administration of medications rather than a nurse or caregiver documenting on a paper chart.
    A. Computer-Physician Order Entry
    B. Electronic Medication Administration Record
    C. E-Prescribing
    D. Direct Entry

22. _____ is the electronic entry of instructions from practitioners in a hospital for patient orders.
    A. Computer-Physician Order Entry
    B. Electronic Medication Administration Record
    C. E-Prescribing
    D. Direct Entry

23. At what temperature should the storage refrigerator in a pharmacy be kept?
    A. 10 - 20°F   B. 20 - 30°F   C. 26 - 36°F   D. 36 - 46°F

24. Which of the following is the process of sending back medications when expired, damaged, or destroyed for credit from manufacturers?
    A. Negative Inventory Event   B. Positive Inventory Event
    C. Reverse Distribution   D. Negative Distribution

25. Which of the following is the amount of stock that should be on the shelves to meet demands and when a drug falls below predetermined quantities it is automatically reordered?
    A. Periodic Automatic Replacement
    B. Pareto Method
    C. Hybrid Cycle Counting Methods
    D. Cycle Counting by Usage

KEY (CORRECT ANSWERS)

1.	B	11.	A
2.	A	12.	B
3.	B	13.	C
4.	C	14.	A
5.	C	15.	C
6.	C	16.	B
7.	C	17.	A
8.	C	18.	B
9.	D	19.	C
10.	C	20.	C

21. B
22. A
23. D
24. C
25. A

EXAMINATION SECTION

TEST 1

DIRECTIONS: Each question or incomplete statement is followed by several suggested answers or completions. Select the one that BEST answers the question or completes the statement. *PRINT THE LETTER OF THE CORRECT ANSWER IN THE SPACE AT THE RIGHT.*

1. Which of the following is NOT necessary in determining the status of a patient's insurance?   1._____
   A. Gender
   B. Marital status
   C. Food preferences
   D. Name of drug plan and identifying numbers

2. The cost of a Glucophage tablet is $200 per 50 tablets. How much would the cost of the prescription be for 60 tablets and the patient is eligible for a 20% senior citizen discount?   2._____
   A. $48   B. $192   C. $220   D. $240

3. Which of the following insurance plans would cover individuals with end-stage renal disease?   3._____
   A. Medicaid   B. Medicare   C. TRICARE   D. CHAMPVA

4. _____ is defined as paying a fixed, pre-paid fee per person to provide a range of health services which is normally paid prior to services being provided.   4._____
   A. Capitation   B. Fee for service
   C. Manage care   D. Self-pay

5. _____ is a set fee that is paid for each type of service that is performed as is paid at the time of service.   5._____
   A. Capitation   B. Fee for service
   C. Manage care   D. Self-pay

6. All of the following are examples of managed care providers EXCEPT   6._____
   A. Health Maintenance Organizations
   B. Preferred Provider Organizations
   C. Exclusive Point of Service
   D. Health Care Indemnity

7. All of the following are characteristics of Health Maintenance Organizations EXCEPT: 7._____
   A. Goal is to keep patients healthy
   B. Capitation reimbursement plan
   C. High flexibility in selection of providers
   D. Primary care physician directs all medical care for members

8. All of the following are characteristics of Preferred Provider Organizations EXCEPT:
   A. Provide health care services to members at a discounted fee for service
   B. Non-exclusive contract with network providers
   C. No co-pay
   D. Members may select a non-PPO provider but must pay the difference

   8.____

9. All of the following are characteristics of a Point of Service Plan EXCEPT:
   A. Members may choose an HMO or PPO for services
   B. May see out-of-network providers
   C. Higher costs for out-of-network providers
   D. Lower premiums

   9.____

10. Which of the following is a characteristic of Exclusive Point of Service Plans?
    A. PPO does not make payments to providers outside the network
    B. Lower premiums
    C. Little flexibility in selection of providers
    D. Proactive health care plan

    10.____

11. Which of the following is a financial account established by an individual/family to pay for qualified medical expenses?
    A. Private plan
    B. Medication Assistance Program
    C. Health savings account
    D. Fee-for-service

    11.____

12. _____ are established by drug manufacturers and other organizations to provide medications to qualified patients who are unable to afford their medications.
    A. Private plan
    B. Medication Assistance Program
    C. Health savings account
    D. Fee-for-service

    12.____

13. _____ is a federal program to provide health care for elderly adults, persons with disabilities, and patients with end-stage renal disease.
    A. Medicare
    B. Medicaid
    C. Medigap
    D. Health Maintenance Organization

    13.____

14. Which part of Medicare covers inpatient hospital care, skilled nursing facilities, hospice, and home health care?
    A. Part A   B. Part B   C. Part C   D. Part D

    14.____

15. Which of the following allows participants in Medicare Part A and Part B to obtain coverage through an HMO or PPO that provides additional services at a higher cost?
    A. Medicaid
    B. Medigap
    C. Medicare Advantage
    D. Exclusive Point of Service

    15.____

16. Which part of Medicare provides for physician services, outpatient care, and some physical and occupational therapy?
    A. Part A	B. Part B	C. Part C	D. Part D

17. Which part of Medicare provides for prescription medications, biologicals, insulin, vaccines, and select medical supplies?
    A. Part A	B. Part B	C. Part C	D. Part D

18. Which of the following is an additional policy that covers areas that are not covered by Medicare?
    A. Medicaid	B. Medigap
    C. Medicare Advantage	D. Exclusive Point of Service

19. _____ is a federal program that is based on income and other circumstances that are determined by each state.
    A. Medicaid	B. Medigap
    C. Medicare Advantage	D. Medicare

20. All of the following are examples of pharmacy provider networks EXCEPT
    A. Point of Service	B. Community Pharmacy
    C. Mail Order	D. Physician Dispensing

21. Which pharmacy provider network consists of both chain pharmacies and independent pharmacies and may be an open or closed network?
    A. In-house network	B. Mail-order pharmacy network
    C. Community pharmacy network	D. Physician dispensing network

22. Which pharmacy provider network consists of a pharmacy owned by an HMO, normally located in an HMO facility, and provides pharmacy services only for members of the network?
    A. In-house network	B. Mail-order pharmacy network
    C. Community pharmacy network	D. Physician dispensing network

23. _____ is the process which enables the use of nonformulary drugs once the physician requests and documents the reason why the medication is needed.
    A. Formulary Override	B. Prior Authorization
    C. Restricted Formulary	D. Exclusive Formulary

24. Which of the following is a six-digit number used to identify the company that will reimburse the pharmacy for the prescription being filled?
    A. Bank Identification Number	B. Plan Code
    C. Group Code	D. Dispense and Written Code

25. Which of the following is used to ensure the pharmacy is properly reimbursed by a third party provider for a prescription being dispensed?
    A. Bank Identification Number	B. Plan Code
    C. Group Code	D. Dispense and Written Code

KEY (CORRECT ANSWERS)

1.	C		11.	C
2.	B		12.	B
3.	B		13.	A
4.	A		14.	A
5.	A		15.	C
6.	D		16.	B
7.	C		17.	D
8.	C		18.	B
9.	D		19.	A
10.	A		20.	A

21. C
22. A
23. B
24. A
25. D

TEST 2

DIRECTIONS: Each question or incomplete statement is followed by several suggested answers or completions. Select the one that BEST answers the question or completes the statement. *PRINT THE LETTER OF THE CORRECT ANSWER IN THE SPACE AT THE RIGHT.*

1. All of the following are situations in which prior authorization would be warranted EXCEPT
   A. expense medications
   B. medications with age limits
   C. drugs used for cosmetic purposes
   D. medications for life-threatening medical conditions

   1.____

2. _____ is defined as the maximum amount of medication that may be dispensed at one time, normally expressed as a day's supply.
   A. Prescription limitations   B. Drug benefit limitations
   C. Dollar limit   D. Prescription cap

   2.____

3. _____ is defined as the maximum number of prescriptions that can be dispensed over a period of time which includes refills and is normally 1 year for non-controlled prescriptions.
   A. Prescription limitations   B. Drug benefit limitations
   C. Dollar limit   D. Prescription cap

   3.____

4. Which of the following is defined as the maximum amount that can be spent per period of time, normally a year?
   A. Prescription limitations   B. Drug benefit limitations
   C. Dollar limit   D. Prescription cap

   4.____

5. Which of the following is defined as the maximum amount that can be spent at one time on a prescription?
   A. Prescription limitations   B. Drug benefit limitations
   C. Dollar limit   D. Prescription cap

   5.____

6. A _____ is a predetermined amount of money that must be spent on a prescription.
   A. deductible   B. dollar limit
   C. prescription cap   D. plan code

   6.____

7. What type of copayment consists of a predetermined dollar amount per prescription filled?
   A. Fixed   B. Percentage   C. Variable   D. Direct

   7.____

8. What type of copayment consists of a different payment based on the type of drug being dispensed in which generic and formulary drugs are encouraged?
   A. Fixed   B. Percentage   C. Variable   D. Direct

   8.____

9. As a general rule, Medicaid reimburses what percentage less than Medicare?
   A. 10% B. 25% C. 40% D. 50%

10. Which of the following has a slightly higher reimbursement rate than Medicare?
    A. Medicaid
    B. Self-pay
    C. Third-party payers
    D. Medigap

11. All of the following are services that can be proved and billed for in the community setting EXCEPT
    A. medication therapy management
    B. immunizations
    C. acute care chart reviews
    D. disease state education services

12. Who requires that medication therapy management services are performed at least once per year?
    A. Medicaid
    B. Medigap
    C. Medicare Part B
    D. Medicare Part D

13. All of the following immunizations can be administered by and billed for by a pharmacy EXCEPT
    A. measles, mumps, rubella
    B. influenza
    C. pneumonia
    D. meningitis

14. Medicare Part B will cover diabetes education for what time period within a 12-month period?
    A. 4 hours B. 8 hours C. 10 hours D. 12 hours

15. Which of the following must pay full price for prescriptions either with cash, check, credit, or debit card?
    A. Medicaid
    B. Self-pay
    C. Third-party payers
    D. Medigap

16. Which of the following is described as a pharmacy submitting prescription claims electronically to a third-party provider when filling a prescription to ensure copayments and timely payment?
    A. E-prescribing
    B. Formulary override
    C. Online adjunction
    D. Prior authorization

17. A _____ is a unique number assigned to health care providers in order to transmit health information according to the health Insurance Portability and Accountability Act?
    A. bank identification number
    B. national provider number
    C. national drug classification number
    D. group code

18. _____ is a government health benefits program for military personnel and retirees which also includes dependents of active-duty service members.
    A. Medicare B. Medicaid C. Tricare D. Champva

19. _____ is a health benefits program that helps pay medical expenses for families of veterans who have been disabled because of injuries related to military experience.
    A. Medicare B. Medicaid C. Tricare D. Champva

20. Which of the following is a third-party administrator of prescription drug programs who processes and pays for all drug claims and manages the formulary for each plan?
    A. Pharmacy Benefit Manager
    B. Pharmacist-in-Charge
    C. Pharmacy Claims Administrator
    D. Pharmaceutical Executive Officer

21. _____ is the process of determining whether or not a drug will be covered under the insurance plan.
    A. Adjunction
    B. Adjudication
    C. Collaboration
    D. Deliberation

22. Patient care supplies such as insulin supplies and nebulizers are classified as which of the following under Medicare Part B?
    A. Outpatient services
    B. Physician services
    C. Hospital services
    D. Durable medical equipment

23. A _____ is the fee that the patient pays at the time of service.
    A. Deductible
    B. Co-insurance
    C. Co-payment
    D. Premium

24. What portion of prescription drug costs do patients pay who are covered by Workers' Compensation?
    A. 0% B. 10% C. 20% D. 25%

25. A _____ is an evaluation required by the Omnibus Budget Reconciliation Act to determine whether a medication is safe for the patient based on selective criteria and cost-effective measures.
    A. compliance report
    B. drug utilization review
    C. ABC analysis
    D. velocity report

KEY (CORRECT ANSWERS)

1.	D		11.	C
2.	A		12.	D
3.	B		13.	A
4.	D		14.	C
5.	C		15.	B
6.	A		16.	C
7.	A		17.	B
8.	C		18.	C
9.	D		19.	D
10.	C		20.	A

21. B
22. D
23. C
24. A
25. B

EXAMINATION SECTION
TEST 1

DIRECTIONS: Each question or incomplete statement is followed by several suggested answers or completions. Select the one that BEST answers the question or completes the statement. *PRINT THE LETTER OF THE CORRECT ANSWER IN THE SPACE AT THE RIGHT.*

1. Which of the following is a large, expensive computer that is powerful enough to process a large quantity of data?
   A. Mainframe computer
   B. Dumb terminals computer
   C. Minicomputer
   D. Microcomputer

   1.____

2. A _____ computer allows multiple users to access patient information.
   A. mainframe
   B. dumb terminals
   C. mini
   D. micro

   2.____

3. All of the following are hardware components of a microcomputer EXCEPT
   A. monitor
   B. central processing unit
   C. printer
   D. operating systems

   3.____

4. Which of the following are smaller scaled mainframes that are used by several people through the use of a local area network?
   A. Mainframe computer
   B. Dumb terminals computer
   C. Minicomputer
   D. Microcomputer

   4.____

5. All of the following are functions of a microcomputer EXCEPT
   A. quality assurance
   B. drug utilization review
   C. adverse drug reports
   D. verify prescriptions

   5.____

6. Components such as the monitor, mouse, and printer are all controlled by which of the following?
   A. Hardware
   B. Softwar
   C. Minicomputers
   D. Microcomputers

   6.____

7. Which of the following governs the operations of the computer?
   A. Operating systems
   B. Central processing unit
   C. Hardware
   D. Microcomputers

   7.____

8. Components such as the keyboard, mouse, trackball, and voice recognition are all considered to be which of the following?
   A. Hardware
   B. Software
   C. Input devices
   D. Software applications

   8.____

9. _____ support pharmacy practices and user desired tasks.
   A. Operating systems
   B. Software applications
   C. Input devices
   D. Central processing unit

10. All of the following are considered to be types of computer output devices EXCEPT
    A. touchscreen   B. speakers   C. printers   D. monitors

11. Which of the following allows the computer to communicate over a network?
    A. Operating systems
    B. Software applications
    C. Modem
    D. Processor

12. _____, also known as RAM, provides a computer with temporary workspace.
    A. Memory   B. Storage   C. Interfaces   D. Processor

13. _____ allows for computer connections between two or more computer systems.
    A. Software applications
    B. Central processing units
    C. Interfaces
    D. Modem

14. Which of the following is the "brains" of the computer workstation?
    A. Operating system
    B. Processor
    C. Keyboard
    D. Monitor

15. Health information technology is used in accordance to standards set by which agency?
    A. Food and Drug Administration
    B. Joint Commission
    C. American Pharmacists Association
    D. American Medical Association

16. All standardized orders and guidelines need to be developed, tested, and approved by the Hospital _____ Committee.
    A. Executive
    B. Safety
    C. Pharmacy and Therapeutics
    D. Ethics

17. Which organization focuses on pharmacy services and developed SCRIPT standards?
    A. National Council for Prescription Drug Programs
    B. Food and Drug Administration
    C. American Pharmacists Association
    D. Pharmacy Services Technical Advisory Coalition

18. In order to obtain federal insurance reimbursement, SCRIPT is a standard that is mandated for medical providers that use
    A. written prescriptions
    B. verbal prescriptions
    C. prescriptions for controlled substances
    D. electronic prescriptions

19. All of the following are included under SCRIPT standards EXCEPT
    A. coding for pharmacy billing and secures a place for electronic data interchange
    B. transfer of prescription data among pharmacies, prescribers, intermediaries, and payers
    C. enhancements for drug use, drug utilization review, signatures, allergies, and diagnosis information
    D. messages regarding new prescriptions, prescription changes, refill requests, prescription cancellation, medical history, and transactions for long-term care facilities

19.____

20. Which organization has established HIPAA compliant current procedural terminology billing codes for pharmacists when doing medical therapy management?
    A. Academy of Managed Care Pharmacy
    B. National Association of Chain Drug Stores
    C. Pharmacy Services Technical Advisory Coalition
    D. American Society of Consultant Pharmacists

20.____

21. Which of the following is a computer-to-computer transfer of prescription data among prescribers, pharmacies, and payers which is an integral step in achieving broad use of electronic health records?
    A. Telepharmacy
    B. E-prescribing
    C. Point of Care
    D. Computerized Physician Order Entry

21.____

22. _____ are a digital, interoperable standard that automates and streamlines clinician's workflow, generates complete record of clinical patient encounter, and includes patient health records such as demographics, progress, mediations, and vital signs.
    A. Electronic health records
    B. Electronic personal health record
    C. Computerized physician order entry
    D. E-prescribing

22.____

23. All of the following statements are true regarding electronic personal health records EXCEPT:
    A. Made by physicians, patients, hospitals, and pharmacies
    B. Controlled by patient or legal proxy and given to health care provider when needed
    C. Automates and streamlines clinician's workflow
    D. Used by pharmacies in providing medical therapy management

23.____

24. Which of the following is a clinical information system that enables the patient's care provider to enter medication orders or a certain procedure into a computer that is transmitted to the appropriate department or individual? 24.____
    A. Electronic health records
    B. Electronic personal health record
    C. Computerized physician order entry
    D. E-prescribing

25. All of the following statements are true regarding computerized physician order entry EXCEPT: 25.____
    A. Can include passwords or fingerprints to sign in
    B. Access from any patient care setting, pharmacy, physician office, or home
    C. Maintains patient data such as allergies, height, weight, current medications, and diagnoses
    D. Place where pharmacist and patient try to address, identify, resolve, and prevent drug-related issues

KEY (CORRECT ANSWERS)

1.	A	11.	C
2.	B	12.	A
3.	D	13.	C
4.	C	14.	B
5.	D	15.	B
6.	B	16.	C
7.	A	17.	A
8.	C	18.	D
9.	B	19.	A
10.	A	20.	C

21. B
22. A
23. C
24. C
25. D

TEST 2

DIRECTIONS: Each question or incomplete statement is followed by several suggested answers or completions. Select the one that BEST answers the question or completes the statement. *PRINT THE LETTER OF THE CORRECT ANSWER IN THE SPACE AT THE RIGHT.*

1. Which of the following is the place where the pharmacist and the patient try to address, identify, resolve, and prevent drug-related issues?
    A. Electronic health records
    B. Electronic personal health record
    C. Computerized physician order entry
    D. Point of care

2. Which of the following is considered to be a DISADVANTAGE associated with e-prescribing?
    A. Creates electronic records
    B. Speeds up refill requests
    C. Transaction fee incurred by the pharmacy
    D. Improves efficiency

3. All of the following statements are true regarding telepharmacy EXCEPT:
    A. Brings the pharmacy to patients when it is not possible for the patient to get to the pharmacy
    B. Provides video conferencing used to give real time counseling
    C. Cost effective method to give pharmacy services
    D. Allows patients better access to medical records

4. All of the following statements are true regarding HIPAA and technology EXCEPT:
    A. HIPAA requires ID or protected health information to be held confidentially
    B. Decreases patient access to medical records
    C. Prescriber order entry complements technology with HIPAA
    D. Patient information is portable and information on the internet can be moved between systems

5. _____ documentation principle ensures all recorded information meets legal, regulatory, institutional policy, and other requirements?
    A. Unique patient ID   B. Accuracy
    C. Completeness   D. Timeliness

6. The _____ documentation principle requires healthcare documentation to occur during or immediately after an event.
    A. unique patient ID   B. accuracy
    C. completeness   D. timeliness

7. The _____ documentation principle enables authorized practitioners to capture, share, and report information from any system.
   A. completeness
   B. timeliness
   C. interoperability access documentation systems
   D. retrievability

8. The _____ documentation principle requires the use of standard titles, formats, templates, abbreviations, terminology, and coding to enable authorized data searches and indexing.
   A. authentication and accountability
   B. auditability
   C. interoperability across documentation systems
   D. retrievability

9. The _____ documentation principle includes devices and systems that create or generate information and takes responsibility for the information accuracy and timeliness.
   A. authentication and accountability
   B. auditability
   C. interoperability across documentation systems
   D. retrievability

10. The _____ documentation principle allows users to examine basic information such as data fields and disclosure of personal health information as well as alerting users of errors, inappropriate changes, and potential security breaches.
    A. authentication and accountability   B. auditability
    C. confidentiality and security   D. retrievability

11. The _____ documentation principle ensures adherence to legislation, regulations, guidelines, and policies through a documentation process as well as alerting users of potential security breaches.
    A. authentication and accountability   B. auditability
    C. confidentiality and security   D. retrievability

12. Which of the following would be a management function performed by ambulatory pharmacy computer systems?
    A. Generating reports
    B. Verifying orders entered by techs
    C. Accessing patient information
    D. Accessing information regarding drug-food interactions

13. All of the following information can be accessed through a clinical decision support system EXCEPT
    A. therapeutic duplication   B. financial reports
    C. drug-allergy interactions   D. IV compatibility

14. All of the following statements are true regarding computer usage to control inventory EXCEPT used to
    A. track costs
    B. monitor purchases and usage
    C. alert to outdated inventory
    D. dispose of outdated inventory

15. All of the following statements are true regarding computer usage and narcotics control EXCEPT:
    A. Maintains narcotic and error discrepancy reports
    B. Maintains reports for daily controlled substance use by patients and quantity
    C. Determines what dose of narcotics to be administered to the patient
    D. Maintains records of expired controlled substances

16. All of the following are advantages to automated ambulatory care systems EXCEPT:
    A. Minimum number of prescriptions to be filled per day to be cost effective
    B. Can count and prefill containers of medications
    C. Provide pharmacist more time to practice clinical skills
    D. Better efficiency and accuracy of prescription filling and dispensing

17. All of the following statements are true regarding ambulatory care automated prescription systems EXCEPT:
    A. Computers can be shared between pharmacies of the same chain
    B. Payer, insurance carrier, and third party billing functions allow for processing of insurance claims
    C. Allows for dispensing medications not covered by insurance plan
    D. Can count and prefill containers of medications

18. Which of the following is the PRIMARY purpose of automated systems?
    A. Reduce medication errors
    B. Count, package, and label dosage forms
    C. Improve documentation
    D. Replace labor intensive tasks

19. Which of the following is a DISADVANTAGE to automated systems in a centralized inpatient pharmacy?
    A. Improved accuracy on bar code recognition
    B. Not all systems can stock items such as injectable, bulk, or refrigerated items
    C. Cost savings on bulk purchasing
    D. Improve efficiency of dispensing functions

20. All of the following are advantages for automated systems in a decentralized inpatient pharmacy EXCEPT:
    A. Dispensing functions in batch mode not on demand
    B. Tracks expiration dates
    C. Cost of equipment and remodeling
    D. Reduces order turnaround time by moving inventory to point of care

21. All of the following information is included in a drug bar code EXCEPT
    A. drug name
    B. dosage form
    C. drug strength
    D. patient name

22. Which of the following is a DISADVANTAGE of using barcodes?
    A. Not every drug is barcoded
    B. Portable and can be used anywhere
    C. Scans NDC# bar code on patient label or receipt and matches it to scanned NDC# on stock drug
    D. Can scan bar code on drug against patient wristband to make sure right drug and dosage given to the right person at the right time

23. Alert _____ is defined as too many alerts going off which can contribute to alerts being ignored.
    A. avoidance
    B. fatigue
    C. overload
    D. ignorance

24. All of the following are risks associated with health information technology EXCEPT:
    A. Patient safety risk during implementations if not carefully planned and followed
    B. Medication errors due to mislabeling of bar codes and unclear/confusing computer screens
    C. Payer, insurance carrier, and third party billing functions allow for processing of insurance claims
    D. Adverse events may occur because of strain of healthcare personnel if workflow becomes complicated

25. Which of the following is a centralized system that uses bar coding technology, a network of computers, a conveyor system, and machines to pick medications according to a patient's profile and place the drug in the correct patient's medication drawer?
    A. Cybernetics
    B. Robotics
    C. Ergonomics
    D. Cyclotronics

KEY (CORRECT ANSWERS)

1. D
2. C
3. D
4. B
5. C

6. D
7. C
8. D
9. A
10. B

11. C
12. A
13. B
14. D
15. C

16. A
17. C
18. B
19. B
20. C

21. D
22. A
23. B
24. C
25. B

EXAMINATION SECTION

TEST 1

DIRECTIONS: Each question or incomplete statement is followed by several suggested answers or completions. Select the one that BEST answers the question or completes the statement. *PRINT THE LETTER OF THE CORRECT ANSWER IN THE SPACE AT THE RIGHT.*

1. The degree to which a drug or other substance becomes available to the target tissue after administration is referred to as
    A. affinity
    B. absorption
    C. bioavailability
    D. solubility

    1.____

2. _____ is the process whereby a drug increases the concentration of certain enzymes that affect the pharmacologic response to another drug.
    A. Absorption
    B. Bioavailability
    C. Induction
    D. Inhibition

    2.____

3. Which of the following blood elements has a protective property against heart disease?
    A. Cholesterol
    B. Triglycerides
    C. Low-density lipoproteins
    D. High-density lipoproteins

    3.____

4. Which of the following would represent common adverse reactions of antiarrhythmic drugs?
    A. Lightheadedness, hypotension, and weakness
    B. Headache, hypertension, and lethargy
    C. Weakness, lethargy, and hyperglycemia
    D. Anorexia, GI upset, and hypertension

    4.____

5. Which of the following represents the BEST definition for hemostasis?
    A. Thinning the blood for better flow in the vessels
    B. Stopping all evidence of bleeding
    C. Forming a clot and stopping bleeding
    D. Forming a clot in the venous circulation

    5.____

6. Which class of drug is used for the prevention of angina pain?
    A. Calcium channel blockers
    B. Nitrates
    C. Beta-adrenergics
    D. Phosphodiesterase inhibitors

    6.____

7. For what reason would parenteral therapy be initiated?
    A. Patient cannot feed themselves
    B. Ease for care providers
    C. Inability to handle GI nutrition
    D. Promote a better outcome for the patient

    7.____

8. An allergy to what food substance would be an indicator of an allergy to the measles vaccine?
   A. Eggs B. Peanuts C. Gelatin D. Wheat

9. Which of the following substances would decrease the absorption of oral iron?
   A. Antacids
   B. Levothyroxine
   C. Ascorbic acid
   D. Vitamin B12

10. Benzodiazepines enhance the function of which neurotransmitter?
    A. Acetylcholine
    B. GABA
    C. Norepinephrine
    D. Serotonin

11. Xanax is contraindicated for a patient with which of the following medical conditions?
    A. Glaucoma
    B. Congestive heart failure
    C. Diabetes
    D. Hypertension

12. Schizophrenia involves an overabundance of which neurotransmitter?
    A. Acetylcholine
    B. Dopamine
    C. Norepinephrine
    D. Serotonin

13. Which of the following is a sign of drug withdrawal and not an adverse reaction?
    A. Dizziness
    B. Metallic taste
    C. Constipation
    D. Sedation

14. DEA Form _____ would be appropriate when contacting the DEA pertaining to theft in a pharmacy?
    A. 106 B. 111 C. 222 D. 224

15. A pharmacy must notify the board in writing if it plans on closing within _____ days.
    A. 7 B. 14 C. 30 D. 60

16. What is the refill limit for C-III to C-V medications?
    A. No refills
    B. 1 refill/90 days
    C. 2 refills/120 days
    D. 5 refills/6 months

17. Which piece of legislation provided a streamline approval process for generic drugs with the creation of the Amended New Drug Application?
    A. Orphan Drug Act
    B. Waxman-Hatch Act
    C. Prescription Drug Marketing Act
    D. Kefauver-Harris Amendment

18. Which piece of legislation draws the distinction between compounding and manufacturing?
    A. Prescription Drug Marketing Act
    B. Prescription Drug User Fee Act
    C. Food and Drug Modernization Act
    D. Orphan Drug Act

19. The United States requires the presence of which food coloring agent to be declared on food and drug products?
    A. Indigotine   B. Erythrosine   C. Tartrazine   D. Amaranth

20. The remainder of a prescription should be filled within _____ after a partial filling.
    A. 24 hours   B. 48 hours   C. 72 hours   D. 7 days

21. Which piece of legislation defines a valid prescription for controlled substances is one issued for a legitimate medical purpose by a practitioner who has conducted at least one in person medical evaluation with the patient?
    A. Prescription Drug Marketing Act   B. Prescription Drug User Fee Act
    C. Food and Drug Modernization Act   D. Ryan Haight Act

22. In what Title of the Code of Federal Regulations are all FDA regulations contained?
    A. 5   B. 12   C. 17   D. 21

23. For what reason did Congress pass the Pure Food and Drug Act of 1906?
    A. Rise in drug trafficking
    B. Birth defects caused by thalidomide
    C. Deaths due to diethylene glycol ingestion
    D. Unsanitary and poorly labeled food and drugs

24. Poor outcomes following the ingestion of _____ led to the adoption of the Kefauver-Harris Amendments of 1962.
    A. Colored food additives   B. Thalidomide
    C. Sulfanilamide   D. Diethylene glycol

25. Which of the following requires FDA approval prior to implementation by the manufacturer?
    A. Label change to strengthen the warnings
    B. Changes in manufacturing
    C. Changes in the way the drug is synthesized
    D. Label change to strengthen dosage information

KEY (CORRECT ANSWERS)

1.	C		11.	A
2.	C		12.	B
3.	D		13.	B
4.	A		14.	A
5.	C		15.	B
6.	A		16.	D
7.	C		17.	B
8.	C		18.	C
9.	A		19.	C
10.	B		20.	C

21. D
22. D
23. D
24. B
25. C

TEST 2

DIRECTIONS: Each question or incomplete statement is followed by several suggested answers or completions. Select the one that BEST answers the question or completes the statement. *PRINT THE LETTER OF THE CORRECT ANSWER IN THE SPACE AT THE RIGHT.*

1. _____ is defined as the process of killing or destroying all microorganisms and their pathogenic products.
   A. Sanitization   B. Disinfection
   C. Sterilization   D. Medical asepsis

   1._____

2. What type of sterilization uses a combination of heat, steam, and pressure to sterilize?
   A. Autoclave   B. Dry heat sterilization
   C. Gas sterilization   D. Chemical sterilization

   2._____

3. Sterile products can be frozen for a time period of
   A. 24 hours   B. 7 days   C. 30 days   D. 45 days

   3._____

4. _____ are sweetened liquids that contain water and alcohol which are made by dissolving alcohol soluble ingredients in ethanol and water soluble ingredients in water, then adding the water to the ethanol under constant stirring.
   A. Suspensions   B. Solutions   C. Elixers   D. Emulsions

   4._____

5. _____ are suspensions made up of either small inorganic particles or large organic molecules that are interpenetrated by a liquid and can work externally or systemically.
   A. Linaments   B. Ointments   C. Creams   D. Gels

   5._____

6. A _____ airflow hood can be used for all chemotherapeutic agents and can also be used to mix non-chemotherapeutic agents.
   A. laminar   B. horizontal   C. vertical   D. diagonal

   6._____

7. _____ is the process of grinding powders to reduced particle size.
   A. Trituration   B. Dilution   C. Spatulation   D. Levigation

   7._____

8. Which of the following are chemicals produced by microorganisms that can cause a fever reaction in patients?
   A. Antigen   B. Pyrogen   C. Pathogen   D. Carcinogen

   8._____

9. If a medication has proven to put a human fetus at risk the risk outweighs the benefit, and the drug should be avoided during pregnancy. This drug belongs to the FDA class of medication called FDA Pregnancy Category
   A. A   B. C   C. D   D. X

   9._____

10. A _____ order is a type of medication generally used on an emergency basis and means the drug is to be administered as soon as possible but only once.
    A. stat   B. single   C. standing   D. PRN

11. The _____ name of a drug is the universally accepted name and considered the official proprietary name for the drug.
    A. chemical   B. generic   C. trade   D. brand

12. Which of the following is defined as a maintained concentration of a drug in the plasma during a series of scheduled doses?
    A. Cumulative effect
    B. Onset of action
    C. Peak plasma level
    D. Plateau

13. Prescriptions for controlled medications must be written on a script pad of what color?
    A. White   B. Pink   C. Green   D. Blue

14. Which of the following is a type of non-preventable medication error?
    A. First time allergy
    B. Wrong patient
    C. Wrong time
    D. Wrong drug form

15. The raised area on the body that indicates a positive response to the tuberculin skin test is referred to as a(n)
    A. induration   B. inunction   C. carbuncle   D. foruncle

16. What type of medications are not regulated by the FDA, should be included in the patient's medical record, and patient should be asked if they are being taken?
    A. Controlled substances
    B. Over-the-counter medications
    C. Herbal supplements
    D. Anabolic steroids

17. Drug _____ is defined as one drug modifying the actions of another drug, may increase or decrease the action of the drug, and may alter the way the drug is absorbed in the body.
    A. interaction   B. response   C. allergy   D. tolerance

18. _____ is defined as conversion of a drug to inactive form and excreted through the GI tract.
    A. Absorption   B. Excretion   C. Metabolism   D. Toxicity

19. What type of medications stimulates the full evacuation of the bowels?
    A. Expectorants   B. Cathartics   C. Toxoids   D. Suspensions

20. Drug _____ is common among the elderly and occurs when medications accumulate in the blood after a prolonged intake of a medication.
    A. toxicity   B. response   C. allergy   D. tolerance

21. What type of facility is NOT certified by the Joint Commission?   21.____
    A. Hospitals   B. Nursing homes
    C. Long-term care facilities   D. Retail pharmacies

22. Which of the following is NOT required on the label of a repackaged   22.____
    medication?
    A. Date of repackaging
    B. Generic name of the medication
    C. Manufacturer's name and lot number
    D. Beyond-use date after repackaging

23. USP _____ is a chapter of the USP which addresses sterile compounding.   23.____
    A. <642>   B. <795>   C. <797>   D. <808>

24. For states requiring that pharmacy technicians be certified, for what period   24.____
    of time is this certification valid?
    A. 1 year   B. 2 years   C. 3 years   D. 5 years

25. _____ alcohol is a type of alcohol which should be used when cleaning   25.____
    pill trays.
    A. Ethyl   B. Isopropyl   C. Methyl   D. Isobutyl

KEY (CORRECT ANSWERS)

1.	C	11.	B
2.	A	12.	D
3.	D	13.	D
4.	C	14.	A
5.	D	15.	A
6.	C	16.	C
7.	A	17.	A
8.	B	18.	C
9.	D	19.	B
10.	A	20.	A

21. D
22. A
23. C
24. B
25. B

TEST 3

DIRECTIONS: Each question or incomplete statement is followed by several suggested answers or completions. Select the one that BEST answers the question or completes the statement. *PRINT THE LETTER OF THE CORRECT ANSWER IN THE SPACE AT THE RIGHT.*

1. How often do pharmacy weights need to be calibrated? 1.____
   A. Weekly B. Monthly
   C. Every 6 months D. Annually

2. What is the MINIMUM number of times a prescription should be viewed when filling a prescription? 2.____
   A. 2 B. 3 C. 4 D. 5

3. What part of the prescription includes the name and strength of the medication prescribed and the amount to be dispensed? 3.____
   A. Inscription B. Sigma C. Subscription D. Superscription

4. DAW _____ is a DAW code that should accompany a medication when a pharmacist requests brand name product be dispensed. 4.____
   A. 0 B. 1 C. 3 D. 5

5. A(n) _____ label is defined as a bright, colorful label placed on a bottle label to provide information in addition to what is on the bottle label and alerts patients to specific information to which careful attention should be paid. 5.____
   A. precaution B. auxiliary C. warning D. instruction

6. The first five numbers in an NDC number represent drug 6.____
   A. manufacturer B. entity C. package D. name

7. If the instruction for a medication is to be taken at bedtime, what abbreviation should be denoted on the prescription? 7.____
   A. am B. bid C. hs D. pm

8. What is the meaning of the abbreviation "au"? 8.____
   A. Each ear B. Left ear C. Right eye D. Each eye

9. How many micrograms are in one grain? 9.____
   A. 32,500 B. 48,750 C. 65,000 D. 81,250

10. How many teaspoon doses are there in a pint of elixir? 10.____
    A. 24 B. 48 C. 72 D. 96

11. Prescribers must use tamper-resistant prescriptions for which group of patients? 11.____
    A. Medicare B. Medicaid C. Elderly D. Adolescent

12. The _____ is the part of the prescription that includes directions to the pharmacist for dispensing the medication.
    A. inscription
    B. signatura
    C. subscription
    D. superscription

13. How many pills should be included in a 30 day prescription to be taken qod?
    A. 15
    B. 30
    C. 60
    D. 120

14. Which of the following is required for metered dose inhalers, oral contraceptives, estrogen, progesterone, and isotretinoin?
    A. MSDS sheets
    B. Patient package inserts
    C. Unit of use container
    D. Beyond use date

15. A(n) _____ order is a medication order given on an "as needed" basis for specific signs and symptoms.
    A. admission
    B. discharge
    C. PRN
    D. STAT

16. A(n) _____ inventory indicates the actual quantity of medication on hand at a particular moment in time.
    A. initial
    B. perpetual
    C. biannual
    D. biennial

17. What must be provided to the purchaser if a pharmacy stocks hazardous materials?
    A. Facts and comparison data sheet
    B. Safety data sheet
    C. Manufacturer's product insert
    D. Patient product insert

18. What is the purpose of a group purchasing organization for a hospital pharmacy?
    A. Negotiate prices with drug manufacturers
    B. Negotiate prices with a local drug wholesaler
    C. Purchase drugs for the hospital from a drug manufacturer
    D. Purchase drugs from a local drug wholesaler

19. A(n) _____ agreement is a type of agreement which is made between a pharmacy and a wholesaler in which the pharmacy agrees to purchase the majority of its product from the wholesaler?
    A. Prime purchaser
    B. prime vendor
    C. exclusive rights
    D. exclusive purchaser

20. Which of the following terms refers to the form to order drugs or supplies from a wholesaler?
    A. Just-in-time ordering
    B. Point of service
    C. Purchase order
    D. Want book

21. Which type of drug would use a drug accountability record?
    A. Over-the-counter medication
    C. Controlled substances
    C. Investigational drugs
    D. Proprietary drugs

22. A Class _____ drug recall is associated with irreversible damage or death to an individual.
    A. I B. II C. III D. IV

23. DEA Form _____ is required to be completed in the destruction of noncontrolled substances.
    A. 41 B. 106 C. 222 D. 224

24. A(n) _____ copayment is a type of copayment which offers a different payment based on the type of drug being dispensed, encourages generic and formulary drugs, and provides greater access of drugs to members but with a higher copay.
    A. fixed B. percentage C. variable D. indemnity

25. A(n) _____ formulary includes a very limited number of drugs with a limited number of medications available in each therapeutic classification.
    A. open B. closed C. restricted D. exclusive

KEY (CORRECT ANSWERS)

1. D
2. B
3. A
4. C
5. B

6. A
7. C
8. A
9. C
10. D

11. B
12. B
13. A
14. B
15. C

16. B
17. B
18. A
19. B
20. D

21. C
22. A
23. A
24. C
25. B

TEST 4

DIRECTIONS: Each question or incomplete statement is followed by several suggested answers or completions. Select the one that BEST answers the question or completes the statement. *PRINT THE LETTER OF THE CORRECT ANSWER IN THE SPACE AT THE RIGHT.*

1. A(n) _____ network includes a pharmacy that is owned by an HMO, normally located in the HMO facility, and provides pharmacy services only for members of the network.
   A. physician dispensing
   B. community pharmacy
   C. in-house
   D. mail-order pharmacy

   1.____

2. Medicare Part _____ is a part of Medicare which provides for prescription medications, biologicals, insulin, vaccines, and select medical supplies.
   A. A
   B. B
   C. C
   D. D

   2.____

3. _____ are established by drug manufacturers and other organizations to provide medications to qualified patients who are unable to afford their medications.
   A. Health savings accounts
   B. Private plans
   C. Medication assistance programs
   D. Coupons

   3.____

4. Which of the following are provided as an incentive for physicians on the original filling of a new prescription in which the value is deducted from what the patient is responsible for paying?
   A. Health savings accounts
   B. Private plans
   C. Medication assistance programs
   D. Coupons

   4.____

5. Which of the following provides healthcare services to members at a discounted fee for service, has a nonexclusive contract with network providers, requires a copay at time of service, and percentage paid by the insurance is lower if services are provided by an out-of-network provider?
   A. Health Maintenance Organization
   B. Preferred Provider Organization
   C. Point of Service Plan
   D. Exclusive Point of Service Plan

   5.____

6. The goal of a(n) _____ is to keep patients healthy, proactive healthcare, has a predictable cost, and offers little flexibility in selection of providers.
   A. Health Maintenance Organization
   B. Preferred Provider Organization
   C. Point of Service Plan
   D. Exclusive Point of Service Plan

   6.____

7. Which of the following patient monitoring functions detects patients on drugs in the same therapeutic classification?
   A. IV compatibility
   B. Drug-drug interaction
   C. Drug-allergy interaction
   D. Drug-laboratory test interaction

   7.____

8. Which of the following is NOT an advantage of centralized automation?
   A. Able to trace expiration dates
   B. Improves accuracy of bar code recognition
   C. Improved inventory management
   D. Located in a patient care unit

   8.____

9. Which of the following statements is TRUE regarding information files on a computer database?
   A. Must be backed up daily
   B. Must be kept separately
   C. Must be kept in a procedure and policy manual
   D. Must be maintained in alphabetical order

   9.____

10. Which of the following statements is TRUE regarding sign-on or access codes?
    A. All pharmacy staff have the same level of security assigned to their access codes
    B. Everyone uses the same code
    C. Sign-ons identify the individual using the code
    D. A technician does not need to sign off before someone else uses the same terminal

    10.____

11. Which of the following is a means to access a pharmacy computer system?
    A. Biometrics
    B. Biometrics and electronic signature
    C. Electronic signature
    D. User name and password

    11.____

12. What principle of documentation uses standardized titles, formats, and templates?
    A. Accuracy   B. Auditability
    C. Confidentiality   D. Retrievability

    12.____

13. Which of the following would NOT be found in database maintenance?
    A. Clinical monitoring   B. Drug files
    C. Patient information   D. Physician files

    13.____

14. _____ brings the pharmacy to patients when the patient is not able to get to the pharmacy. Video conferencing is used to provide real time counseling and is a cost-effective method to provide pharmacy services.
    A. E-prescribing   B. Point of care services
    C. Telepharmacy   D. Virtual Pharmacy

    14.____

15. Which of the following is considered to be a DISADVANTAGE regarding e-prescribing? 15._____
    A. Reduces prescription errors
    B. Creates electronic health records
    C. Transaction fee incurred by the pharmacy
    D. Speeds up refill requests

KEY (CORRECT ANSWERS)

1.	C	6.	A	11.	D
2.	D	7.	B	12.	D
3.	C	8.	D	13.	C
4.	D	9.	A	14.	C
5.	B	10.	C	15.	C

INTRODUCTION TO PHARMACY

Section I. GENERAL

Purpose and scope. This manual provides guidance and information for pharmacy specialists. It will supplement instructions given in pharmacy classes and in organized on-the-job training programs and will serve as a reference for basic procedures performed by pharmacy personnel.

Section II. HISTORY, ETHICS, AND REFERENCES OF PHARMACY

History of Pharmacy
a. Derivation of names.

(1) The word "pharmacy" is derived from the Greek pharmakon, which originally meant "a charm," later "a poison," and finally "a drug." Pharmacy and medicine were professions of great mystery in early times. Disease was at first believed to be a manifestation of the presence of evil spirits in the body. To drive away these evil spirits, the physicians of ancient times employed a series of rituals consisting of chants, noises, ceremonies, and odors.

(2) Aesculapius, son of Apollo, was the Roman and Greek god of healing. The staff of Aesculapius, represented by a staff branched at the top with a snake entwined around it, is used as a symbol of medicine and as the official insignia of the American Medical Association. (It should not be confused with the caduceus, the "Herald's Wand," used by Hermes, or Mercury, which shows two serpents on a staff mounted by wings.)

b. Papyrus Ebers. Among early documents dealing with pharmacy and medicine is the Papyrus Ebers, dating from about the 16th century BC, or shortly before the time of Moses. (This scroll is named for Georg Moritz Ebers, 1837-1898, German Egyptologist, who edited the medical papyrus which he had discovered in Thebes.) This manuscript is a continuous roll more than 250 feet long and about a foot wide. It contains information about 700 remedies for afflictions, methods of compounding, and ways of conjuring away diseases. It indicates that diagnosis had been highly developed as an art for some time at this early period; some of the drugs it mentions are still in common use.

c. Hippocrates. Hippocrates, a Greek physician who was born on the Island of Cos in 460 BC, is called the "Father of Medicine." His fame is based largely on his assumed authorship of the Hippocratic Oath, which he exacted from his students. Some authorities, however, believe the oath was written after Hippocrates' death. This oath, still taken by modem physicians, is a code of conduct for the medical profession. Hippocrates taught the "humoral theory" of disease, which proposed that improper balance of the four humors of medieval physiology-blood, phlegm, yellow bile, and black bile-caused disease.

d. Galen. At the beginning of the Christian era, several Greeks and Romans were noted in medicine. Galen (131-201 AD), a Greek who became a Roman citizen, originated so many vegetable drugs by mixing and melting individual ingredients that these preparations are still called "galenical preparations" or "galenicals." Galen's Cerate is still synonymous for the term "cold cream," a preparation which he originated nearly 2000 years ago.

e. Pharmacy as a science. The beginning of the Crusades in the 11th century had a stimulating effect upon all areas of scientific and professional knowledge. Pharmacy was taught as part of the curricula of medicine in schools of this period.

(1) A decree of the German Emperor Frederick II in 1240 contains the first undoubted record of the separation of medicine and pharmacy. This edict regulated the practice of pharmacy in his kingdom of the two Sicilies. Under this regulation, physicians were neither allowed to operate pharmacies nor to realize any profit from selling medicine by clandestine arrangements with apothecaries. The management and responsibilities of these pharmacies were restricted and they were allowed only in principal cities.

(2) Toward the end of the 12th century, one of the first organized bodies of pharmacists came into existence in Florence as part of the guild of physicians and apothecaries.

(3) In the 16th century, Philippus Aureolus Theophrastus Bombastus von Hohenheim, Swiss physician and alchemist (1493-1541), advanced ideas about the internal use of chemicals in treating diseases, and was instrumental in the development of pharmaceutical chemistry. He is best known by the name "Paracelsus." His work greatly changed the train of thought in the medical field.

f. Pharmacopeias. A pharmacopeia is an official book of standards for drugs. Pharmacopeias are very valuable to physicians and pharmacists. The first official book of standards listing drugs for chemical use was issued in 1613. It was the sixth edition of the Pharmacopoeia of Augsburg, known as the Pharmacopoeia Augustana. Soon after this came the fust London Pharmacopoeia of 1618, the frrst pharmaceutical book of standards which was mandatory for an entire nation. Later, Scotland, Ireland, Germany, and the United States published similar works.

g. Modern pharmacy practice. Since these historic periods, the practice of pharmacy – insofar as its external appearances are concerned – has changed considerably, but it is still chiefly involved in the compounding, dispensing, and selling of remedial agents.

h. History of pharmacy in America.

(1) Even before Europeans arrived on the soil which now makes up the United States, scores of herbs were used as therapeutic agents by the Indians in this country. Some are still recognized in The United States Pharmacopeia and The National Formulary. Among the herbs that the Indians used were blackberry, cascara sagrada, dandelion, dogwood, elderberry, juniper, podophyllum, raspberry, senega, slippery elm, tobacco, white pine, wild cherry, wintergreen, and witch hazel.

(2) During the 17th century, pharmacy and medicine in America were closely identified with members of sectarian movements arriving in this country. Each group exerted its influence upon the nation's pharmacy and medicine by introducing the scientific knowledge and remedies its members had brought from their homeland. Throughout this century, the American housewife took over most of the medical care of her family and was often the only source of medical information available; this medical information was handed down from generation to generation.

(3) In the 18th century, the filling of prescriptions written by medical practitioners flourished into a specialized art. This prepared the way for the recognition of the profession of pharmacy as distinct from the profession of medicine. In 1775, the Continental Congress established the first Army hospital; the first military apothecary, Andrew Craigie, was on its staff.

(4) A definite trend toward the development of scientific and professional pharmacy was evident during the 19th century. Many pharmaceutical associations came into being. In 1817, South Carolina enacted the first legislation making an examination and a license prerequisites to the practice of pharmacy. Organized professional pharmacy began with the founding of the Philadelphia College of Pharmacy in 1822. In rapid sequence, several other colleges of

pharmacy were formed. During the 1800's, many notable figures of modem pharmacy exerted their influence. Some of the best-known men in this category were Joseph P. Remington, Eli Lilly, E. R. Squibb, Charles Dohme, and Frederick Steams. The American Pharmaceutical Association (A.Ph.A.), founded in 1852, set down a code of ethics similar to that of the Philadelphia College of Pharmacy.

(5) In the present century, the Federal Food and Drugs Act of 1906 recognized The United States Pharmacopeia and The National Formulary as the basis for drug standards. A revised Federal Food, Drug, and Cosmetic Act, enacted in 1938, established many new regulations. The Harrison Narcotic Act was passed into law in 1914 and limited the sale of opium and its derivatives. It required registration of all individuals and firms engaged in the purchasing, processing, compounding, and sale of narcotic drugs.

(6) Pharmacy in the Armed Forces is not new. Before World War II, enlisted men were responsible, under the supervision of physicians, for the pharmacy function. In 1943, legislation provided for the formation of a Pharmacy Corps, and licensed pharmacists of the Regular Army Medical Administration Corps automatically became members. The Pharmacy Corps was designated by insignia of a caduceus with a superimposed letter "P." In 1947, the Medical Service Corps of the Regular Army was established which absorbed the Pharmacy Corps. In today's Army, pharmacies are under the control of a pharmacy officer, who is a graduate, licensed pharmacist, except in rare cases where no commissioned officer who is a pharmacist is on duty. (This can occur when the unit's TOE does not contain a slot for such an officer. In this case, the duties of the pharmacy officer are assigned to a Medical Corps officer.) The pharmacies and dispensaries in the Army are further manned by additional pharmacy officers, plus enlisted personnel who are registered pharmacists or military trained pharmacy specialists. They all work under the control and supervision of the Chief, Pharmacy Service.

Pharmacy ethics. The term "ethics" is defined as the standards of conduct for a profession. It is a moral code by which the members of a profession must abide. Below are excerpts from the accepted Code of Ethics of the American Pharmaceutical Association:

a. Obligation. "The primary obligation of pharmacy is the service it can render to the public in safeguarding the preparation, compounding, and dispensing of drugs, and the storage and handling of drugs and medicinal supplies."

b. Knowledge, skill, and integrity. "The practice of pharmacy requires knowledge, skill, and integrity; therefore, the state laws restrict the practice of pharmacy to persons with special training."

and qualiflcations and license to them privileges which are denied to others. Accordingly, the pharmacist recognizes his responsibility to the state and to the community for their well-being, and fulftlls his professional obligations honorably."

c. The pharmacist and his relations to the public.

(1) "The pharmacist upholds the approved legal standards of The United States Pharmacopeia and The National Formulary, and encourages the use of official drugs and preparations. He purchases, compounds, and dispenses only drugs of good quality."

(2) "The pharmacist uses every precaution to safeguard the public when dispensing any drugs or preparations. Being legally entrusted with the dispensing and sale of these products, he assumes this responsibility by upholding and conforming to the laws and regulations governing the distribution of these substances."

(3) "The pharmacist seeks to enlist and to merit the confidence of his patrons. He zealously guards this confidence. He considers the knowledge and confidence which he gains of the ailments of his patrons as entrusted to his honor, and does not divulge such facts."

(4) "The pharmacist keeps his pharmacy clean, neat, and sanitary, and well-equipped with accurate measuring and weighing devices and other apparatus suitable for the proper performance of his professional duties."

(5) "The pharmacist holds the health and safety of his patrons to be of first consideration; he makes no attempt to prescribe for or to treat disease or to offer for sale any drug or medical device merely for profit."

(6) "The pharmacist is a good citizen and upholds and defends the laws of the states and nation; he keeps informed concerning pharmacy and drug laws, and other laws pertaining to health and sanitation, and cooperates with the enforcement authorities."

(7) "The pharmacist supports constructive efforts in behalf of the public health and welfare. He seeks representation on public health committees and projects and offers to them his full cooperation."

d. The pharmacist in his relations to other health professions.

(1) "The pharmacist willingly makes available his expert knowledge of drugs to the other health professions."

(2) "The pharmacist refuses to prescribe or to diagnose; he refers those needing such service to a properly licensed practitioner. In an emergency and pending the arrival of a qualified practitioner, he applies such first aid treatment as is dictated by humanitarian impulses, scientific knowledge, and good judgment."

(3) "The pharmacist compounds and dispenses prescriptions carefully and accurately, using correct pharmaceutical skill and procedure. If there is any question in the pharmacist's mind regarding the ingredients of a prescription, a possible error, or the safety of the direction, he privately and tactfully consults the practitioner before making any changes. He exercises his best professional judgment and follows, under the laws and existing regulations, the prescriber's directions in the matter of refilling prescriptions, copying the formula upon the label, or giving a copy of the prescription to the patient. He adds any extra directions or caution or poison labels only with proper regard for the wishes of the prescriber, and the safety of the patient

(4) "The pharmacist does not discuss the therapeutic effects or composition of a prescription with a patient. When such questions are asked, he suggests that the qualified practitioner is the proper person with whom such matters should be discussed."

e. The pharmacist and his relations to fellow pharmacists.

(1) "The pharmacist strives to perfect and enlarge his professional knowledge. He contributes his share toward the scientific progress of his profession and encourages and participates in research, investigation, and study. He keeps himself informed regarding professional matters by reading current pharmaceutical, scientific, and medical literature, attending seminars, and other means."

(2) "The pharmacist seeks to attract to his profession youth of good character and intellectual capacity and aids in their instruction."

(3) "The pharmacist associates himself with organizations having for their objective the betterment of the pharmaceutical profession and contributes his share of time, energy, and funds to carry out the work of these organizations."

(4) "The pharmacist keeps his reputation in public esteem by continuously giving the kind of professional service that earns its own reward. He does not engage in any activity or transaction that will bring discredit or criticism to himself or to his profession."

(5) "The pharmacist will expose any corrupt or dishonest conduct of any member of his profession which comes to his certain knowledge, through those accredited processes provided by the civil laws or the rules and regulations of pharmaceutical organizations, and he will aid in driving the unworthy out of the calling."

(6) "The pharmacist does not lend his support or his name to the promotion of objectionable or unworthy products."

(7) "The pharmacist courteously aids a fellow pharmacist who may request advice or professional information."

(8) "The pharmacist is proud to display in his establishment his own name and the names of other pharmacists employed by him."

NOTE

Although this code of ethics was written for the graduate, registered pharmacist, it contains basic doctrine and moral guidelines for all who deal with pharmacy. Stand by this code at all times and your career will be a pleasant one for you, for the men serving with you, and for the patients you assist.

Compendia, references, and reference library. Pharmacy and its allied fields are so complex that one cannot hope to learn and retain all the data necessary for all situations. For this reason, every pharmacy must have a reference library of well-selected books such as those mentioned below. Having or acquiring the reference library is the first step; the second step is using it.

a. Official pharmacy references. There are two official books used by the pharmacist. They are The Pharmacopeia of the United States of America (commonly known as The United States Pharmacopeia or USP) and The National Formulary (NF). These are the pharmaceutical standards made official by the Food and Drugs Act of 1906 which was rewritten and re-enacted by Congress in 1938. It was amended in 1951 and 1962 and is now entitled the Food, Drug, and Cosmetic Act.

(1) The United States Pharmacopeia (USP). The USP is an authoritative book on drugs and their preparation. In it is a list of accepted medical drugs and chemicals, with descriptions of each; tests; purities; formulas; and average doses. The USP first appeared in 1820 and is now revised and published every 5 years by the United States Pharmacopeial Convention. This convention is made up of delegates from the professions of medicine, dentistry, pharmacy, and chemistry. The USP is restricted to drugs and preparations which have stood the test of modem research and continued use. Since agents are accepted by the USP only after continued

successful use, the newest ones are often excluded. The monographs, that is, the explanations of the individual preparations, contain the following information:

(a) *Official English titles.* Example: calcium hydroxide.

(b) *Botanical names* (for plant drugs). Example: Atropa belladonna.

(c) *Symbolic formulas* (in the case of chemicals). Example: Ca (OH)2.

(d) *Structural formulas* (in the case of organic chemicals whenever the formula is generally accepted by chemists). Example: aspirin.

[Structural formula of aspirin: benzene ring with CO CH and O-CO-CH3 substituents]

(e) *Official definitions.* In order that no question shall arise as to the exact meaning of an official title, the USP states exactly what kind or variety of the substance should be used. Example: Acacia. "Acacia is the dried gummy exudate from the stems and branches of Acacia senegal (Linne) Willdenow or of other related African species of Acacia (Fam. Leguminosae)."

(f) *Purity rubric.* This term indicates the paragraph limiting the quantity of impurity allowed by giving the percentage of pure substance that must be present. Example: Aspirin. "Dry it over silica gel for 5 hours: It loses not more than 0.5 percent of its weight."

(g) *Official description.* This description usually consists of a concise statement of the drug's physical properties and appearance. Example: Aspirin occurs as "White crystals, commonly tabular or needle-like, or white, crystalline powder. Is odorless or has a faint odor. Is stable in dry air; in moist air it gradually hydrolyzes to salicylic and acetic acids."

(h) *Tests for purity and identity.* In the USP, the tests which establish the identity of a drug and those which insure the pharmacopeial minimum degree of purity are grouped under appropriate headings.

(i) *Assays.* Chemicals, preparations, and certain crude drugs have assays included in their monographs which are intended to insure their contents to be in accord with the "purity rubric."

(j) *Packaging and storage.* Certain official drugs and preparations have packaging and storage directions listed under the title of the same name. These specifications are intended to maintain the activity and potency of the drug or preparation for a maximum period. Example: Alcohol. "Preserve in tight containers, remote from fire."

(k) *Preparations available.* When the pharmacopeial substance is used in the manufacture of other pharmacopeial preparations, these preparations are usually listed. *Example:* Aminophylline."Suppositories usually available contain the following amounts of aminophylline: 100, 125,250, and 500 mg."

(l) Labels. If special labels are required, notations will generally be made in italicized print, but these may be made under the speciftc title of labels.

(m) Category. The drug is classified into groups according to its therapeutic use and action. Example: Aspirin. "Category: Analgesic; antipyretic; antirheumatic."

(n) Dose. The dose is given in the metric system. It is listed as the usual dose, the range of dosage possible without harmful effects, and the method or route of administration. Example: Aspirin.

"Usual Dose: Oral or rectal, 600 mg. 4 to 6 times a day as necessary.

Usual Dose Range: Oral, 300 mg. to 8 grams daily. Rectal, 300 mg. to 2 grams daily."

(2) The National Formulary (NF). The purpose of *The National Formulary* is to supply legal standards for drugs and formulations commonly used in medical practice which may not have been recognized for medical efficiency by the USP, but which have had long and customary use. The NF is much the same as the USP in arrangement. It, too, is revised and issued at S-year intervals to coincide with the USP schedule. It is pu blished by the American Pharmaceutical Association through its committee on the National Formulary.

b. Important nonofficial references. Besides the two official books already described, there are many other texts which are of great assistance to the pharmacist. The following books are not official, but are recognized as being standard references.

(1) United States Dispensatory (USD). The *United States Dispensatory* expands broadly on the USP and NF, adding information such as unofficial synonyms, pharmacology, toxicology, and dosage schedules.

(2) Pharmaceutical Recipe Book. The Pharmaceutical Recipe Book provides formulas for preparations not found in the official books which are frequently required in hospitals and pharmacies.

(3) Merck Index. The Merck Index contains listings of over 8000 chemicals and drugs, and information about each.

(4) New Drugs (ND). The ND is published by the Council on Pharmacy and Chemistry of the American Medical Association. It lists and describes the drugs that have been accepted by the council. The descriptions of the accepted drugs are based, in part, on evidence of information supplied by the manufacturer. Statements made by those commercially interested are critically examined and the drug is admitted only when such statements are supported by other evidence or when they conform to known facts. Drugs in the ND often have not been used in practice long enough to be admitted to The United States Pharmacopeia.

(5) Merck Manual. The Merck Manual essentially provides condensed medical information. It lists diseases, causes, prevention, treatment, prescriptions, prognoses, diagnoses, etc.

(6) Modern Drug Encyclopedia and Therapeutic Index. The book contains information on proprietary drugs (patented, trademarked medicinals) supplied by their manufacturer.

(7) Remington's Pharmaceutical Sciences. The "Remington," as it is most frequently called, is an excellent and most complete reference to the overall picture of pharmacy.

NOTES AND RESOURCES
CONTENTS

	Page
I - GLOSSARY OF DRUGS WITH NATIONAL NOMENCLATURES	
Anesthetics	1
Muscle Relaxants	1
Narcotics	2
Hypnotics	2
Antibiotics	2
Drugs Affecting Sympathetic Nervous System and Nerve Endings	3
Electrolytes	3
Plasma Expanders	4
Miscellaneous Drugs	4
Vaccines and Antitoxins	5
Antiseptics	5

II - USEFUL TABLES

		Page
Table 1.-	Atomic Weights, Valences, and Equivalent Weights of Certain Elements	6
Table 2.-	Milliequivalent Per Gram of Certain Elements and Compounds	6
Table 3.-	Normal Range of Concentration of Serum Constituents	6
Table 4.-	Normal Range of Concentration of Whole Blood Gases and pH Values	6
Table 5.-	Equivalent United States and Imperial Weights and Measures	7
Table 6.-	Approximate Equivalent Metric and Imperial Doses	7
Table 7.-	Equivalent Avoirdupois and Metric Weights	8
Table 8.-	Equivalents of Centigrade and Fahrenheit Thermometric Scales	9

NOTES AND RESOURCES

I - Glossary of Drugs With National Nomenclatures
ANESTHETICS

United States	Germany	Netherlands	France
Chloroprocaine N.F	....	Chloroprocaine	
Cocaine hydrochloride U.S.P.	Cocainhydrochlorid DAB 7....................	Cocaine hydrochloride	Cocaine chlorhydrate.
Cyclopropane U.S.P	....	Cyclopentaan	Cyclopropane.
Droperidol	Dehydrobenzperidol	Droperidol	Haldol.
Ether U.S.P	Aether pro narcosi DAB 7 ..	Ether U.S.P.............	Ether pur pour anesthesie.
Halothane U.S.P	Halothan	Halothaan	Halothane.
Lid.ocaine hydrochloride .... U.S.P.	Lidocainii hydrochloridum .... Ph. Int.	Lidocaine hydrochloride	Xylocaine.
Mepivacaine hydrochloride .... N.F.	Scandicain...............	Mepivacaine hydrochloride.	
Nitrous oxide U.S.P .	Distickstoffoxide, Lachgas	Lachgas, distikstofoxide...................	Protoxyde d"azote.
Prilocaine hydrochloride .... N.F.	....	Prilocaine hydrochloride................	
Procaine hydrochloride .... U.S.P.	Procainhydrochlorid DAB 7.	Procaine hydrochloride.	Lignocaine.
Proparacaine hydrochloride .... U.S.P.	....	Proparacaine hydrochloride, ... proxymetacaine.	
Tetracaine hydrochloride .... U.S.P:	Tetracainhydrochlorid DAB 7.	Tetracaine hydrochloride	Tetracaine.
Thiopental sodium U.S.P.	Trapanal	Thiopental-natrium..	Penthiobarbital injectable.

MUSCLE RELAXANTS

United States	Germany	Netherlands	France
Curare	....	Curare.	
Pancuronium bromide	....	Pancuronium bromide.	
Succinylcholine U.S.P	Suxamethonium chloridum .... Ph.Int.	Succinylcholine	Succinylcholine.
Tubocurarine chloride U.S.P.	D-Tubocurarini chloridum Ph.Int.	Tubocurarine chloride	Tubocurarine.

NARCOTICS

Codeine phosphate U.S.P	Codeinphosphate DAB 7...	Codeine fosfaat	Codeine.
Meperidine hydrochloride U.S.P.	Pethidini hydrochloridum Ph.Int.	Pethidine hydrochloride.	Pethidine chlorhydrate.
Methadone hydrochloride U.S.P.	Methadoni hydrochloridum Ph.Int.	Methadon hydrochloride.	
Morphine sulfate U.S.P	Morphini sulfas Ph.Int.....	Morfine sulfaat..	Morphine.
Papaverine hydrochloride .... N.F.	Papaverinhydrochlorid DAB 7.	Papaverine hydrochloride	Papaverine.

HYPNOTICS

Amobarbital U.S.P...	Amobarbitalum Ph.Int.....	Amobarbital	Amobarbital.
Paraldehyde U.S.P..	Paraldehyd DAB 7	Paraldehyde	Paraldehyde.
Pentobarbital U.S.P.	Neodorm.......................	Pentobarbital	Nembutal.
Phenobarbital U.S.P	Phenylaethylbarbitursaure DAB 7.	Fenobarbital	Phenobarbital.
Secobarbital U.S.P..	....	Secobarbital	Secobarbital.

ANTIBIOTICS

United States	Germany	Netherlands	France
Ampicillin U.S.P.......	Amblosin, Binotal.....	Ampicilline	Ampicilline. ....
Bacitracin U.S.P.	Bacitracin	Bacitracine	Bacitracine.
Carbenicillin............	Anabactyl	Carbenicilline.	
Cephaloridine	....	Cefaloridine............	Cephaloridine.
Cephalothin U.S.P ...	Cefalotin	Cefalotine	CepHalotine........
Chloramphenicol U.S.P	Chloramphenicol DAB 7....................	Chlooramfenicol	Chloramphenicol.
Colistin N.F.............	Colistin	Colistine	Colistine.
Erythromycin U.S.P .	Erythromycinum Ph. Int.	Erythromycine	Erythromycine.
Gentamicin sulfate U.S.P....................	Refobacin	Gentamicine sulfaat	Gentamycine.
Kanamycin U.S.P	Kanmytrex, Kanamycin, ... Resistomycin.	Kanamycine	Kanamycine.
Lincomycin U.S.P	Cillimycin	Lincomycine.	
Methicillin U.S.P	Cinopenil	Methicilline	Methicilline.
Neomycin sulfate U.S.P	Neomycin, Bykomycin	Neomycine sulfaat .	Neomycine.
Oxacillin U.S.P.........	Cryptocillin, Stapenor	Oxacilline	Oxacilline.
Polymyxin B sulfate U.S.P...	Polymyxini B-sulfas Ph.Int..	Polymyxine B sulfaat	Polymyxine B.

Potassium penicillin G, ... U.S.P.	Penicillin G-Kalium DAB 7.	Kalium penicilline B ...	Penicilline.
Potassium phenoxymethyl .... penicillin U.S.P.	Beromycin, Immunocillin, ... Isocillin, Aracil.	Kalium fenoxymethyl penicilline.	
Streptomycin sulfate U.S.P., ...	Streptomycinsulfat DAB 7..	Streptomycine sulfaat.	Streptomycine sulfate.
Tetracycline U.S.P ...	Tetracyclinum Ph.Int.	Tetracycline	Oxytetracycline.

DRUGS AFFECTING SYMPATHETIC NERVOUS SYSTEM AND NERVE ENDINGS

Atropine sulfate U.S.P	Atropinsulfat DAB 7	Atropine sulfaat	Atropine sulfate.
Cyclopentolate hydrochloride U.S.P.	....	Cyclopentolaat hydrochloride.	
Epinephrine U.S.P	Adrenalin DAB 7	Adrenaline	Adrenaline. .....
Homatropine hydrobromide U.S.P.	Homatropinhydrobromid .... DAB 7.	Homatropine hydrobromide.	Homatropine bromhydrate.
Isoproterenol U.S.P	Isoprenalini hydrochloridum Ph.Int.	Isoprenaline	Isuprel, isoprenaline.
Levarterenol bitartrate U.S.P.	Noradrenalinhydrogentartrat .... DAB 7.	Levarterenol bitartraat.	Noradrenaline.
Physostigmine salicylate U.S.P.	Physostigminsalicylat DAB 7	Fysostigmine salicyclaat...............	
Pralidoxime chloride U.S.P..	Pralidoximi methiodidum .... Ph.Int.	Pralidoxime chloride	Pralidoxime.
Scopolamine U.S.P	Scopolaminhydrobromid DAB 7.	Scopolamine U.S.P	Scopolamine.

ELECTROLYTES

Calcium gluconate injection .... U.S.P.	Calcium gluconicum 10%	Calcium gluconaat injectie.	Calcium levulinate.
Dextrose injection U.S.P	Traubenzuckerlösung 10%	Glucose injectie	Solution injectable de glucose, isotonique.
Lactated Ringer's injection .... U.S.P.	Ringer-Lactat-Lösung	Ringer lactaat injectie	Lactate de calcium.

| Ringer's injection U.S.P. | Ringer-Lösung............ | Ringer injectie. | Solution de Ringer. |
| Sodium chloride injection .... U.S.P. | Natriumchloridlösung, isotonisch, pyrogen- frei, steril (DAB 7). | Natrium chloride injectie. | Solution inject- able de chlorure de sodium, isotonique. |

PLASMA EXPANDERS

United States	Germany	Netherlands	France
Normal human serum albumin U.S.P.	Humanalbumin 20%	Normal humaan albumine uit serum.	Albumine humaine.
Plasma protein frac- tion U.S.P.	PPL, Humanalbumin 5%.................	Protein fractie uit plasma...........	Gamma globuline.

MISCELLANEOUS DRUGS

United States	Germany	Netherlands	France
Acetylsalicyclic acid U.S.P	Acetylsalicylsaure DAB 7	Acetylsalicyl zuur ..	Acetylsalicylique acide.
Amyl nitrite N.F		Amyl nitriet	Nitrite d'amyle.
Chlorpromazine U.S.P	Chlorpromazini hydro- chloridum Ph.Int.	Chloor promazine	Chlorpromazine.
Digitalis U.S.P	Digitalisblatter DAB 7	Digitalis	Digitaline.
Digoxin U.S.P..........	Digoxinum Ph.Int	Digoxine.	
Ethacrynic acid U.S.P		Ethacryne zuur.	
Furosemide U.S.P...	Lasix	Furosemide	Furosemide- Lasilix.
Hydrocortisone sodium succinate injection U.S.P.	Hydrocortisonhemisuc cinat	Hydrocortison natrium .... succinaat injectie.	Hydrocortisone hemisuccinate.
Mafenide	Marfanil	Mafenide.	
Mannitol U.S.P	D-Mannit	Mannitol.	
Oxygen U.S.P	Sauerstoff	Zuurstof	Oxygene.
Petrolatum U.S.P.	Paraffinum solidum DAB 6, Paraffinum durum DAB 7.	Vaseline	Vaseline.
Probenecid U.S.P ...	Benemid	Probenecide.	
Silver nitrate U.S.P .	Silbernitrat DAB 7 ..	Zilvernitraat	Nitrate d'argent.
Sodium nitrite U.S.P	Natriumnitrit DAB 7.	Natrium nitriet	Nitrite de sodium.
Sodium polysterene sulfonate U.S.P.	Kationen-Austaus- cherharz	Natrium polystyreen sulfonaat.	
Sodium thiosulfate U.S.P.	Natriumthiosulfat DAB 7	Natrium thiosulfaat	Hyposulfite de sodium.

VACCINES AND ANTITOXINS

Gas gangrene antitoxin, pentavalent.	Gasoedem- Antitoxin, polyvalent.	Gas gangreen-antitoxine pentavalent.	Serum antigangreneux polyvalent. ....
Tetanus immune globulin (human) U.S.P.	Tetanus-Immunglobulin	Tetanus-immuno globuoline (menselijk).	
Tetanus toxoid U.S.P.	Tetatoxoid	Tetanus vaccin .	Vaccin antitetanique.

ANTISEPTICS

Alcohol U S P	Aethanol DAB 7	Alcohol	Alcool ethylique.
Hexachlorophene U.S.P	Hexachlorophen WHO	Hexachlorophene .	Exophene.

II - Useful Tables

TABLE 1.— *Atomic weights, valences, and equivalent weights of certain elements*

Element	Atomic weight	Valence	Equivalent weight
Sodium	23.0	1	23.0
Potassium	39.0	1	39.0
Magnesium	24.0	2	12.0
Calcium	40.0	2	20.0
Chlorine	35.5	1	35.5
Phosphorus	31.0	3	10.3
Sulfur	32.0	2	16.0

TABLE 2. *Milliequivalent per gram of certain elements and compounds*

Element or compound	Mini-equivalent	Element or compound	Mini-equivalent
Sodium	43.5	Potassium chloride:	
Potassium	26.0	Potassium	13.5
Magnesium	85.0	Chloride	13.5
Calcium	50.0	Sodium lactate:	
Chloride	29.0	Sodium	9.0
Sodium chloride:		Lactate	9.0
Sodium	17.0		
Chloride	17.0		

364

TABLE 3. *Normal range of concentration of serum constituents*

Constituent		Concentration per 100-milliliters	Milliequivalent per liter
Sodium	milligram	310-340	135-148
Potassium	do	13.6-20.7	3.5-5.3
Magnesium	do	1.8-3.0	1.5-2.5
Calcium	do	9.6-11.0	4.8-5.4
Chloride	do	348-383	98-108
Urea nitrogen	do	8-26	
Carbon dioxide		101-132	23-30 mM
Total protein	gram	6.0-8.2	
Albumin	do	3.8-5.0	
Globulin	do	2.3-3.5	

TABLE 4. *Normal range of concentration of whole blood gases and pH values*

Constituent	Concentration
pO_2 Arterial	90-100 torr[1]
Venous	30 torr
pCO_2 Arterial	35-16 torr
Venous	38-49 torr
pH	7.35-7.45

[1] One torr = 1 mm Hg at sea level.

TABLE 5. *Equivalent United States and imperial weights and measures*

Unit of measurement	Abbreviation	United States measure	Imperial measure
1 milligram	mg	0.015432 grain	0.015432 grain.
1 gram	g	15.432 grains	15.432 grains.
1 kilogram	kg	35.274 ounces (avoirdupois) 32.150 ounces (apothecary)	35.274 ounces (avoirdupois) 35.274 ounces (apothecary).
1 grain	gr	0.0648 gram 64.8 milligrams	0.0648 gram. 64.8 milligrams.
480 grains	gr	31.1035 grams	31.1035 grams.
1 ounce	oz	437.5 grains 28.350 grams	437.5 grains. 28.350 grams.
1 milliliter	ml	16.23 minims	16.894 minims.
1 liter	l	33.814 fluid ounces	35.196 fluid ounces.
1 minim	min	0.0616 milliliter	0.0592 milliliter.
1 fluid ounce	fl oz	29.573 milliliters	28.412 milliliters.
1 pint[1]	Pt	473.17 milliliters	568.25 milliliters.

[1] Sixteen fluid ounces, U.S. measure; 20 fluid ounces, imperial measure.

USEFUL TABLES

TABLE 6. *Approximate equivalent metric and imperial doses*

Milliliters	Minims	Grams	Grains	Milligrams	Grains
0.1	1½	0.1	1½	0.1	1/600
0.12	2	0.12	2	0.125	1/480
0.15	2½	0.15	2½	0.25	1/240
0.2	3	0.2	3	0.3	1/200
0.25	4	0.25	4	0.5	1/120
0.3	5	0.3	5	0.6	1/100
0.4	6	0.4	6	1	1/60
0.5	8	0.5	8	1.5	1/40
0.6	10	0.6	10	2	1/30
1	15	1	15	2.5	1/24
1.3	20	1.3	20	3	1/20
2	30	2	30	5	1/12
3	45	3	45	8	1/8
4	60	4	60	9	3/20
5	75	5	75	10	1/6
6	90	6	90	12	1/5
8	120	8	120	16	1/4
10	150	10	150	20	1/3
15	225	15	225	25	2/5
20	300	20	300	30	1/2
25	375	25	375	50	3/4
				60	1
				75	1 1/4

TABLE 7. *Equivalent avoirdupois and metric weights*

Pounds	Kilograms	Pounds	Kilograms
100	45.359	155	70.306
105	47.627	160	72.574
110	49.895	165	74.842
115	52.163	170	77.110
120	54.431	175	79.378
125	56.698	1 80	81.646
1 30	58.966	185	83.914
1 35	61.234	190	86.182
140	63.502	195	88.450
145	65.770	200	90.718
150	68.038		

TABLE 8. *Equivalents of centigrade and Fahrenheit thermometric scales*

Degrees C	Degrees F	Degrees C	Degrees F	Degrees C	Degrees F
-10	14.0	31	87.8	72	161.6
-9	15.8	32	89.6	73	163.4
-8	17.6	33	91.4	74	165.2
-7	19.4	34	93.2	75	167.0
-6	21.2	35	95.0	76	168.8
-5	23.0	36	96.8	77	170.6
-4	24.8	37	98.6	78	172.4
-2	26.6	38	100.4	79	174.2
-2	28.4	39	102.2	80	176.0
-1	30.2	40	104.0	81	177.8
0	32.0	41	105.8	82	179.6
1	33.8	42	107.6	83	181.4
2	35.6	43	109.4	84	183.2
3	37.4	44	111.2	85	185.0
4	39.2	45	113.0	86	186.8
5	41.0	46	114.8	87	188.6
6	42.8	47	116.6	88	190.4
7	44.6	48	118.4	89	192.2
8	46.4	49	120.2	90	194.0
9	48.2	50	122.0	91	195.8
10	50.0	51	123.8	92	197.6
11	51.8	52	125.6	93	199.4
12	53.6	53	127.4	94	201.2
13	55.4	54	129.2	95	203.0
14	57.2	55	131.0	96	204.8
15	59.0	56	132.8	97	206.6
16	60.8	57	134.6	98	208.4
17	62.6	58	136.4	99	210.2
18	64.4	59	138.2	100	212.0
19	66.2	60	140.0	101	213.8
20	68.0	61	141.8	102	215.6
21	69.8	62	143.6	103	217.4
22	71.6	63	145.4	104	219.2
23	73.4	64	147.2	105	221.0
24	75.2	65	149.0	106	222.8
25	77.0	66	150.8	107	224.6
26	78.8	67	152.6	108	226.4
27	80.6	68	154.4	109	228.2
28	82.4	69	156.2	110	230.0
29	84.2	70	158.0		
30	86.0	71	159.8		

BASIC FUNDAMENTALS OF THE PRESCRIPTION

CONTENTS
Page

SECTION I : PRESCRIPTION LANGUAGE-PHARMACEUTICAL LATIN

1.	Latin in pharmacy and medicine	1
2.	Commonly used Latin abbreviations, words, and translations	1
3.	Common names of drugs and the Latin counterpart	3

SECTION II : THE PRESCRIPTION 3

4.	Superscription	3
5.	Inscription	3
6.	Subscription	4
7.	Signa (signatura)	4
8.	Abbreviation of names of drugs	4
9.	Abbreviation in subscription and signa	4
10.	Prescription examples	4
11.	Importance of pharmaceutical calculations	6
12.	Fractions	7
13.	Rules applying to all fractions	7
14.	Working with fractions	8
15.	Lowest terms	8
16.	Lowest common denomincator (LCD)	8
17.	Adding fractions	9
18.	Subtracting fractions	9
19.	Multiplying fractions	10
20.	Dividing fractions	11
21.	Decimals	12
22.	Adding decimals	12
23.	Subtracting decimals	13
24.	Multiplication of decimals	13
25.	Division of decimals	13
26.	Roman numerals	14
27.	Weights and measures	14
28.	Metric system	15
29.	Apothecary system	17
30.	Avoirdupois system	21
31.	Relationship and approximate equivalents	21
32.	Ratio and proportion	22
33.	Percentage preparations	23
34.	Ratio preparations	25
35.	Specific gravity	26
36.	Specific gravity of liquids	26
37.	Specific gravity of solids	28
38.	Application of specific gravity to pharmaceutical Problems	29
39.	Specific volume	31
40.	Density	31
41.	Temperature	31
42.	Temperature calculation	32
43.	Temperature conversion	32
44.	Dosage	33
45.	Concentration and dilution	36
46.	Alligation	36

BASIC FUNDAMENTALS of the PRESCRIPTION

Section I. PRESCRIPTION LANGUAGE–PHARMACEUTICAL LATIN

1. Latin in pharmacy and medicine. Latin in prescription writing is centuries old. Although more and more of the prescription is being written in English today, most prescriptions are in part written in Latin or use the Latin abbreviations. As long as physicians continue to use Latin and Latin abbreviations in prescription writing, the pharmacist will have to be able to read and fully understand the terms that are used. Latin used in medicine and prescription writing may be intended to conceal the nature of the medication from the patient, to reduce the possibility of a patient's tampering with a prescription, or to make the prescription universally legible to pharmacists regardless of their national language. Probably the most outstanding reason for the use of Latin in medicine and pharmacy is through force of habit. It has been done for so long that it is hard to break away from the trend. Medical and pharmacy colleges teach the physician to write prescriptions in Latin and the pharmacist to be able to interpret them.

2. Commonly used Latin abbreviations, words, and translations. Since it would be extremely time consuming and of doubtful value to present an entire course in Pharmaceutical Latin here, it is strongly suggested that you read, learn, and *memorize* the words, abbreviations, and meanings on the right. This will familiarize you with the more common terms and phrases used in prescription writing and enable you to understand the physician's or other prescriber's orders. Later, when you have time and a desire to improve your command of Latin, as pertinent to pharmacy, procure a copy of an authoritative pharmacy text. With the aid of such a text, the average individual may become familiar with Latin as it applies to the professions of medicine and pharmacy.

Latin	Abbreviation	English Translation
ad	ad	to; up to
ad libitum	ad lib.	at pleasure
adde, addendus	add.	add, let them be added
agitata ante usum	agit. ant. us.	shake before using
albus	alb.	white
alternus horis	alt. hor.	alternate hours
amplus	amplus	large
ana	aa.	of each
ante	a.	before
ante cibos; ante cibum	a.c.	before meals; before food
ante meridiem	A.M.	before noon
applicandus	applicand.	to be applied
aqua	aq.	water
aqua bullions	aq. bull.	boiling water
aqua destillata	aq. dest.	distilled water
aqua fervens	aq. ferv.	hot water
aqua frigida	aq. frig.	cold water
aqua forte	aq. fort.	nitric acid
aromaticus	arom.	aromatic
argentum	arg.	silver
aurio	aur.	ear
bene	ben.	well
bibe	bib.	drink
bis in die	b.i.d.	twice a day
bolus	bol.	a large pill
capeat	cap.	let him take
capsula	cap.	a capsule
charta	chart.	paper (powder)
charta cerati	chart. cerat.	waxed paper
cibus	cib.; c.	food
cochleare amplum	coch. amp.	tablespoonful
cochleare infans	coch. inf.	teaspoonful
cochleare magnum	coch. mag.	tablespoonful
cochleare maximum	coch. max.	tablespoonful
cochleare medium	coch. med.	dessertspoonful
cochleare minimum	coch. min.	teaspoonful
cochleare modicum	coch. mod.	dessertspoonful
cochleare parvum	coch. parv.	teaspoonful
cochleare paulus	coch. paul.	teaspoonful
cochleare plenum	coch. plen.	tablespoonful
cola, colatus	col.	strain, strained
collunarium	collun.	nasal douche
collutorium	collut.	mouthwash
collyrium	collyr.	eye lotion
compositus	comp.	compound,

Latin	Abbreviation	English Translation	Latin	Abbreviation	English Translation
		compounded	misce	M.	Mix
congius	cong.	gallon	mistura	mist.	mixture
continuentur remedia	cont. rem.	continue the medication	mitte	mitt.	send
			modo praescripto	mod. praes.	in the manner prescribed
creta	cret.	chalk			
cum	c.; c̄	with	mollis	moll.	soft
da	d.	give	nasus	n.	nostril
decem	decem	ten	nebula	nebul.	a spray
dentur	dent.; d.	let be given; give	niger	nig.	black
dentur tales doses	d.t.d.	give of such doses	nocte	noct.	at night
dexter	dext.	right			
dies	d.	day	nocte maneque	noct. maneq.; n. et m.	night and morning
diebus alternis	dieb. alt.	on alternate days			
diebus secundis	dieb. secund.	every second day	non	non	not
diebus tertiis	dieb. tert.	every three days	non repetatur	non rep.	do not repeat
diluo; dilutus	dil.	dilute	octarius	O.; oct.	a pint
dispensa; dispensatur	disp.	dispense; let be dispensed	oculus	ocul.	the eye
			oculo dextro	O.D.; ocul. dext.	the right eye, in the
dividatur	div.	divide	oculo sinistro	O.S.; ocul. sinist.	the left eye, in the
dividatur in partes aequales	div. in par. aeq.	divide into equal parts	oculo laevo	O.L.; ocul. laev.	the left eye, in the
			oculo utro	O.U.; ocul. utro	in each eye
dosis	dos.; d.	a dose	oleum	ol.	oil
drachma	ʒ	a drachm	omnis	omn.	every
dura	dur.	hard	omni altera hora	omn. alt. hor.	every alternate hour
e	e	out of; in			
et	et	and	omni hora	omn. hor.	every hour
e lacte	e lact.	in milk	omni mane	omn. man.	every morning
ex modo praescripto	e.m.p.	in the manner prescribed	omni quarta hora	omn. 4 hor.	every four hours
			parvus	parv.	small
fac; fiat; fiant	ft.	make; let be made	per	per	by means of
ferrum	ferr.	iron	per os	per os	by mouth
filtra	filtra	filter	phiala	phial.; p.	a bottle
flavus	flav.	yellow	phiala fusca	phial. fusc.	a brown bottle
folium; folia	fol.	leaf; leaves	phiala prius agitata	p.p.a.	the bottle first being shaken
fortis; fortior	fort.	strong; stronger			
gargarisma	garg.	a gargle	placebo	placebo	I please
gradatim	grad.	gradually	plumbum	plumb.	lead
grossus	gros.	large	ponderosus	pond.	heavy
gramma	Gm.	gram	post aurum	post aur.	behind the ear
granum	gr.	grain	post cibum; post cibos	p.c.	after food; after meals
gutta; guttae	gtt.	drop; drops			
hora	hor.; h	an hour	post meridiem	P.M.	afternoon
hora somni	h.s.	at bedtime	praecipitatus	ppt.	precipitated
hydrargyrum	hydrarg.	mercury	pro capillis	pro capil.	for the hair
in aurem sinistram	in aur. sinist.	in the left ear	pro recto	pro rect.	rectal
			pro re nata	p.r.n.	as occasion arises
in die	in d.	in a day	pro usu externo	pro us. ext.	for external use
in dies	ind.	daily	pulvis	pulv.	powder
in oculo laevo	in ocul. laev; O.L.	in the left eye	quantitatim sufficientum	q.s.	a sufficient quantity
inter	inter	between			
inter cibos	int. cib.	between meals	quaque	qq.	each, every
inter noctem	int. noct.	during the night	quaque die	q.d.	every day
in vitro	in vit.	in glass	quaque hora	q.h.	every hour
lac	lac	milk	quater in diem	q.i.d.	four times a day
levis	lev.	light	repetatur	rep.	let it be repeated
libra	lb.	pound	recipe	Rx; ℞	take thou
liquor	liq.	liquid; solution	ruber	rub.	red
lotio	lot.	lotion	scrupulus	℈	scruple
luteus	lut.	yellow	secundum artem	s.a.	according to the art
magnus	mag.	large	secundum legem	s.l.	according to law
mane	man.	morning, in the	semi	sem.	one-half
massa	mass.	a mass	semissem	ss	one-half
milligramma	mg.; mgm.	a milligram	sesqui	sesqui	one and a half
minimum	♏	a minim			

Latin	Abbreviation	English Translation
signa	sig.; S.	write
simul	simul	at one time
sine	s̄	without
sine aqua	sin. q.; s̄ aq.	without water
si opus sit	s.o.s.	if there is need
solve	solv.	dissolve
spiritus frumenti	sp. frum.	whiskey
spiritus vini rectificatus	S.V.R.	alcohol
spiritus vini tenuis	S.V.T.	diluted alcohol
spiritus vini vitis	sp. vin. vit.	brandy
statim	stat.	immediately
succus	suc.	juice
syrupus	syr.	syrup
tabella	tab.	tablet
talis	tal.; t.	of such
ter in die	t.i.d.	three times a day
tres; trium	tres; trium	three
tussis	tuss.	cough
uncia	℥	ounce
unguentum	ung.; ungt.	ointment
ut dictum	ut dict.	as directed
viridis	vir.	green

3. Common names of drugs and the Latin counterpart

Common Name	Latin
Acid	Acidum
Alcohol	Spiritus Vini Rectificatus (SVR)
Belladonna Leaf	Belladonna Folium
Belladonna Root	Belladonna Radix
Bitter	Amari
Cascara	Rhamnus Purshiana
Castor Oil	Oleum Ricini
Charcoal	Carbo
Wood Charcoal	Carbo Ligni
Clove Oil	Oleum Caryophylli
Coal Tar	Pix Carbonis
Coal Tar Solution	Liquor Carbonis Detergens; Liquor Picis Carbonis
Cod Liver Oil	Oleum Morrhuae
Corn Oil	Oleum Maydis
Cottonseed Oil	Oleum Gossypie Seminis
Earth	Terra
Hard Soap	Sapo Duris
Juice	Succus
Lard	Adeps
Lime	Calx
Linseed Oil	Oleum Lini
Medicinal Soft Soap	Sapo Mollis Medicinalis
Oil	Oleum
Ointment	Unguentum
Orange	Aurantium
Peppermint	Mentha Piperita
Peppermint Oil	Oleum Menthal Piperitae
Purified Cotton	Gossypium Purificatum
Rosin	Resina
Seed	Semen
Sherry Wine	Vinum Xericum
Solution	Liquor
Spearmint Oil	Oleum Menthae Viridis
Spermaceti	Cetaceum
Starch	Amylum
Sucrose	Surcrosum; Saccharum
Sweet	Dulcis
Syrup	Syrupus
Turpentine	Terebinthinae
Wax	Cera
Wild Cherry	Prunus Virginiana
Whiskey	Spiritus Frumenti
White Ointment	Ungunentum Alba
White Wax	Cera Alba
Wool Fat	Adeps Lanae
Yellow Ointment	Unguentum Flavum
Yellow Wax	Cera Flava

Section II. THE PRESCRIPTION

The word prescription is a derivation of two Latin words; namely, "prae," meaning "before," and "scribo," meaning "I write." Therefore, the prescription is something written beforehand, hence a rule or direction. It is a written order to the pharmacist by a physician, dentist, veterinarian, or other licensed practitioner, instructing him to compound and/or dispense a specific medication for a specific patient. Through common misuse, the word prescription has also come to mean the completed medication itself. The completed prescription is generally divided into four subdivisions: Superscription, Inscription, Subscription, and Signa. These four parts, in addition to the patient's name, address, and age; the date of writing; and the prescriber's signature, address, and registry number, make up the correct completed prescription.

4. **Superscription.** The superscription is that which is written above. The superscription always consists of, and is in fact represented by the symbol R_x. This symbol is most frequently printed as part of the prescription blank. R_x is taken from the Latin "recipe," meaning "take thou." It is also thought that the slash across the "R" is a sign for Jupiter and is a carry-down of an invocation to the god.

5. **Inscription.** The inscription, or what is written within, contains the actual ingredients and their respective amounts. Each ingredient is placed on a separate line, and all important words are

capitalized. Quantities are written, as will be seen in section III (Pharmaceutical Calculations), in either the metric or the apothecary system. In the apothecary system, the amount is shown by a symbol followed by a roman numeral, e.g., ℥ viii (eight ounces). In the metric system, a symbol is not used, grams or milliliters being written or understood. The inscription may be further subdivided into base, adjuvant, corrective, and vehicle.

   a. Base. The base is the main or active ingredient or ingredients designed to restore the patient to health.

   b. Adjuvant. The adjuvant is a substance which increases the efficiency of the base.

   c. Corrective. The corrective modifies or counteracts any undesirable effects of the base or adjuvant.

   d. Vehicle. The vehicle may serve several purposes. It may give proper dosage form (producing a liquid, suppository, capsule, etc.). It may dilute so that the patient may take one capsule or one teaspoonful rather than a few grains or a few drops. It may be used to improve taste or appearance. Or it may aid the patient in receiving the proper amount of a potent drug.

6. **Subscription.** The subscription, or that written below, follows the inscription. It tells the pharmacist the manner of compounding and what the finished product shall be. For example: *M. Fiant solutio* means to mix and let a solution be made. The order of the ingredients on the prescription is not necessarily the order in which they are incorporated into the medication. This is up to the pharmacist and is done according to the art of pharmacy. As you will see later in the course, order of mixing has a pronounced effect on many prescriptions and can be the cause of incompatibilities.

7. **Signa (signatura).** The signa follows the subscription and means literally to write. It tells the pharmacist the directions to the patient which will be typed on the label. An example of a signa is: ʒ i t. i. d. Since most individuals have no idea of the meaning of a drachm (ʒ), it must be changed to its approximate equivalent, one teaspoonful. The label would then read: "Take one teaspoonful three times a day." Prescriptions should bear exact instructions to the patient as in figure 2-1 rather than the overused "ut dict," which means "as directed." When directions are specified exactly, there is no doubt that the patient understands how much of the medication he is to take, and at what intervals. Also, by using the directions, the pharmacist is able to check more accurately for excessive dosage. Study figure 2-1 to see the relationship of the superscription, the inscription and its parts, the subscription, and the signa.

8. **Abbreviations of names of drugs.** In writing a prescription, it is always desirable that the official names of agents be used and spelled out completely. Abbreviations or chemical symbols are confusing and can lead to serious error. An abbreviation such as Hyd. Chlor. is not clear. It could be taken for chloral hydrate, for calomel (mercurous chloride), or for mercuric chloride. Chloral hydrate is a hypnotic, used to induce sleep. Calomel is a purgative. Mercuric chloride is a deadly poison even in the smallest doses, and is intended for use as an antiseptic in external preparations to be used on inanimate objects. You can readily see what would happen if one agent were mistaken for another! Imagine the possibilities of confusion with $HgCl$ and $HgCl_2$. $HgCl$ is calomel, the purgative; $HgCl_2$ is mercuric chloride, the poison.

9. **Abbreviations in subscription and signa.** The more important abbreviations for use in the subscription and the signa are given on the preceding pages.

10. **Prescription examples.** Read each of the prescriptions shown in figure 2-2 in English and try to pick out the prescription parts previously described in the text and shown in figure 2-1. Note that the prescriptions in figure 2-2 are written in longhand and use abbreviations. This is the form in which you will most likely see them in the pharmacy.

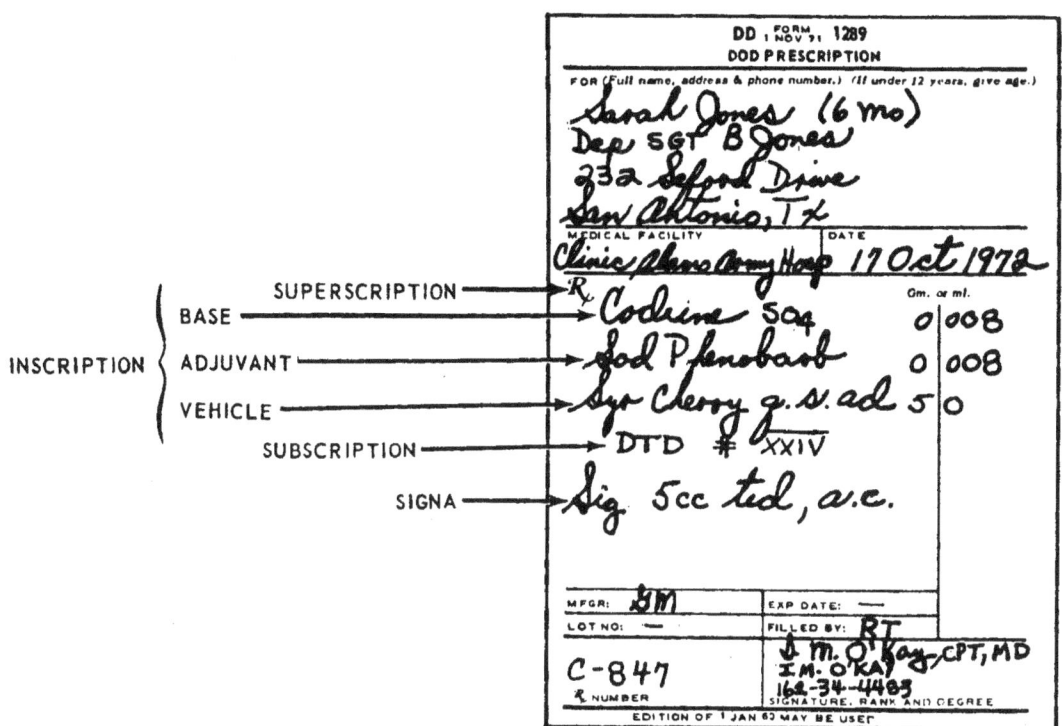

Figure 1. *Components of a prescription.*

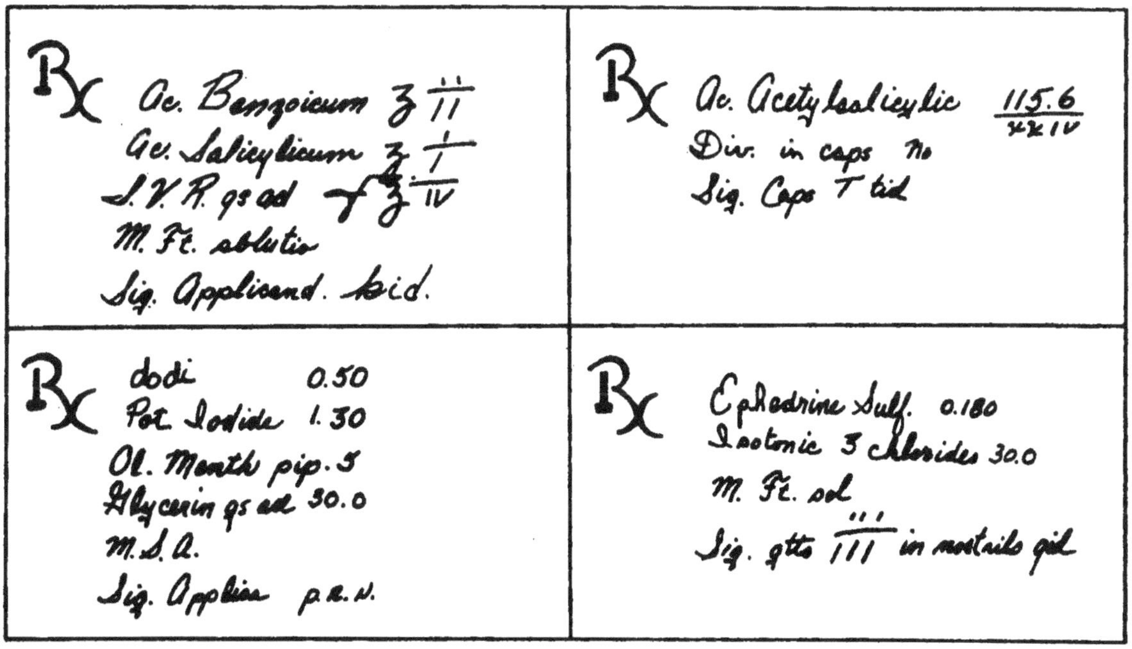

Figure 2. *Prescription examples.*

Section III. PHARMACEUTICAL CALCULATIONS

11. Importance of pharmaceutical calculations. Perhaps the most important and basic study to the pharmacist is the arithmetic and calculations pertinent to prescriptions. Without a complete understanding of the mathematics of pharmacy, the pharmacist is unable to dispense many of the prescriptions and compounds which he is called upon to manufacture. Following are examples of prescriptions and drug orders which you are apt to encounter in your duties as pharmacy technician. By carefully examining the illustrations in figures 2-3 and 2-4, and the text that supports them, you will realize just how important this chapter is to your becoming qualified to manufacture and dispense medicinals.

a. Example of calculations involved in a prescription. In the prescription illustrated by figure 2-3, the physician has specified that each 5 ml. of medication is to contain 0.008 Gm. (8 mg.) each of codeine sulfate and phenobarbital sodium. He further specifies that you are to dispense 24 doses of this completed medication. How much codeine sulfate, phenobarbital sodium, and cherry syrup will you use in compounding this preparation? What will the total volume of the completed prescription be and what size bottle will be used to contain it? Are the doses of each ingredient safe for this 6-month-old child? When you have completed this chapter, you will readily be able to arrive at the answer: 192 mg. each of codeine sulfate and phenobarbital sodium, and enough cherry syrup to make the product measure 120 ml. are necessary in compounding this prescription correctly. The total volume of the completed prescription will be 120 ml. and will be dispensed in a 4-ounce bottle. The doses are safe for this patient. In addition, you will know that the label for this medication should direct that one teaspoonful be given 3 times a day before meals.

b. Example of calculations involved in a bulk order. Figure 2-4 shows a bulk order for an instrument sterilizer solution. The pharmacist has to calculate how much concentrated benzalkonium chloride solution will be necessary to make 4000

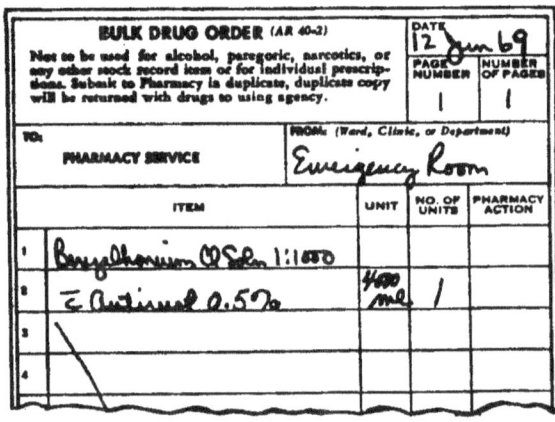

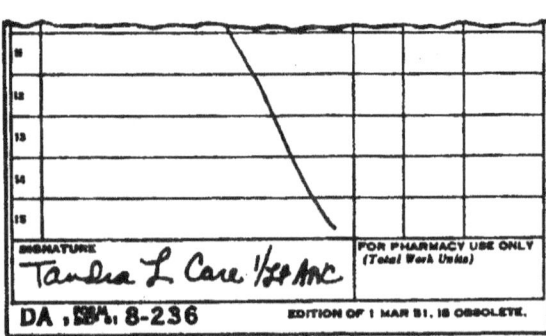

Figure 3. Example of calculations involved in a prescription.

Figure 4. Example of calculations involved in a bulk order.

ml. of a 1:1000 dilution. He will also have to be able to calculate the number of grams of antirust to be used to obtain a 0.5 percent concentration. Upon completing this chapter, it will not be difficult for you to calculate the necessary quantities as being 40 ml. of 10-percent benzalkonium chloride concentrate and 20 Gm. of antirust to make up 4000 ml. of finished solution. These have been but two examples of the absolute necessity of a sound understanding of pharmaceutical arithmetic in pharmacy. As you progress through this chapter, many more will be illustrated and solved.

c. Ground work for pharmaceutical calculations. At first the material that is forthcoming may seem juvenile to you, and you may be inclined to skip over some of the basic aspects. DON'T! Mistakes occur every day in simple addition, subtraction, multiplication, and division. Have you ever caught yourself making such an error? Well, in some places, errors can be allowed for and are not of too much significance, but in pharmacy there is no place for error. First, then, before delving in to the new material, let's begin with a review of fractions and decimals. Here is the place to check yourself on your work. If you work all the problems in fractions and decimals presented in the next few pages, you are well on your way to success in pharmaceutical calculations.

12. **Fractions.** A fraction represents a simple division problem. It expresses one or more of the equal parts into which a whole number is divided. The fraction $\frac{4}{5}$, then, means five divided into four equal parts of a possible five.

a. Numerator. The number above the separating line is called the numerator. It tells how many parts of the whole are used. In our example $\frac{4}{5}$, four parts of the whole are used.

b. Denominator. The denominator is the number below the separating line and represents the number of parts into which the whole is divided. Again using $\frac{4}{5}$ as an example, the whole (1) is broken into five equal parts, four of which remain.

c. Mixed numbers. Numbers made up of a whole number plus a fraction are called mixed numbers. For example, $1\frac{4}{5}$ has the whole number, 1, and the fraction, $\frac{4}{5}$, and is consequently a mixed number. It means that we have a whole of 1, plus 4 of the 5 parts of another whole.

d. Proper fractions. A fraction having a numerator which is smaller than its denominator is a proper fraction. It always is less than a whole number. Again, $\frac{4}{5}$ is a proper fraction.

e. Improper fractions. A fraction having a numerator larger than or equal to its denominator is an improper fraction, and it is always equal to or greater than a whole number. For example, $\frac{5}{4}$ is an improper fraction. It is the same as $1\frac{1}{4}$ ($\frac{5}{4} = \frac{4}{4}$ and $\frac{1}{4}$; $\frac{4}{4} = 1$).

f. Relative values of fractions. Let's compare the relative values of several fractions. Of $\frac{1}{5}, \frac{1}{6}, \frac{1}{3}$, and $\frac{1}{4}$, the smallest is $\frac{1}{6}$. Thus, if fractions have the same numerator, but different denominators, the one with the largest denominator is the smallest in value. Comparing $\frac{2}{5}, \frac{3}{5}$, and $\frac{4}{5}$; the largest is $\frac{4}{5}$. Thus, in fractions having the same denominator but different numerators, the one with the largest numerator is the largest. To compare fractions with different numerators and different denominators is more difficult.

13. **Rules applying to all fractions.** Fractions are division problems and follow three basic rules—

a. Value of fractions maintained. If the numerator and denominator are both multiplied or divided by the same number, the value of the fraction is *not* changed. *Example:* Multiplying both the numerator and denominator of $\frac{1}{3}$ by 3, you get $\frac{3}{9}$ which equals $\frac{1}{3}$; $\frac{3}{9}$ divided by 3 (both numerator and denominator) equals $\frac{1}{3}$ which is equal to $\frac{3}{9}$.

b. Multiplying the value of fractions. If the numerator is multiplied or the denominator divided by a number, the value of the fraction is *multiplied* by that number. *Example:* Multiplying the numerator of $\frac{1}{3}$ by 3 you have $\frac{3}{3}$ which is three times as large; or if you divide the denominator of $\frac{3}{3}$ by 3 you have $\frac{1}{1}$ or 1, which is three times as large.

c. Dividing the value of fractions. If the numerator is divided or the denominator multiplied by a number, the value of the fraction is divided by that number. *Example:* Dividing the numerator of $\frac{3}{9}$ by 3 you have $\frac{1}{9}$, or by multiplying the denominator of $\frac{3}{9}$ by 3 you have $\frac{3}{27}$ which is also $\frac{1}{9}$.

14. Working with fractions. When working with fractions, you often have to reduce a whole number to an improper fraction or reduce an improper fraction to a whole or mixed number.

   a. Reducing a whole or mixed number to an improper fraction.
   (1) Whole number reduction. To reduce a whole number to an improper fraction, it is necessary to know into how many parts you want to divide the whole (the denominator). If you wish to convert 6, for instance, to an improper fraction having 5 parts, you will have 5 as the denominator. If you reduce 1 to an improper fraction having 5 parts, you would have $\frac{5}{5}$. The whole number, 6, when converted to an improper fraction with 5 as the denominator, would be 6 times as large, or $\frac{5}{5} \times 6 = \frac{30}{5}$.

   (2) Mixed number reduction. A mixed number is handled in the same manner. To reduce $8\frac{2}{10}$ to 10ths: $1 = \frac{10}{10}$; then $\frac{10}{10} \times 8 = \frac{80}{10}$ and $\frac{80}{10}$ plus the original $\frac{2}{10} = \frac{82}{10}$, the number of 10ths in $8\frac{2}{10}$.

b. Reducing an improper fraction to a whole or mixed number. As previously stated, a fraction is simply a division problem. For this reason, by dividing the denominator into the numerator, you will get a whole number if the division is even, or a mixed number (whole number plus a remaining fraction) if the division is not even. *Example:* Reduce $\frac{20}{2}$: $\frac{20}{2} = 20 \div 2 = 10$, a whole number; or reduce $\frac{35}{4}$: $\frac{35}{4} = 35 \div 4 = 8\frac{3}{4}$, a mixed number.

15. Lowest terms. A fraction is said to be in its lowest terms when the numerator and denominator cannot be divided by the same number. To illustrate: $\frac{3}{9}$, $\frac{6}{27}$, and $\frac{9}{36}$ are NOT in their lowest terms, for both the numerator and denominator can be divided by a common number. The 3 and 9 in $\frac{3}{9}$ can each be divided by 3 to give $\frac{1}{3}$ which is the lowest terms; the 6 and 27 in $\frac{6}{27}$ by 3 to give $\frac{2}{9}$, the lowest terms; and the 9 and 36 in $\frac{9}{36}$ by 9 to give $\frac{1}{4}$, the lowest terms. These final numbers, then, $\frac{1}{3}$, $\frac{2}{9}$, and $\frac{1}{4}$ are fractions in their lowest terms.

16. Lowest common denominator (LCD). When you add, subtract, or compare fractions, it is necessary to have them in common terms. As apples cannot be added to oranges or automobiles to airplanes, fractions with different denominators cannot be added. By changing apples and oranges to fruit, their common denominator, they can be added. This is also true of fractions. The common denominator can be found by two methods: by multiplying the denominators together, and by a "visual method."

   a. Multiplying denominators to find a common denominator. When all the different denominators of the fractions with which you are dealing are multiplied together, the resulting number is common to all. It is not, however, always the lowest number common to all. For example, to find a denominator common to $\frac{1}{4}, \frac{1}{3}$, $\frac{1}{2}, \frac{1}{8}$, and $\frac{1}{16}$: Multiply the denominators (all of which are different)— 4 x 3 x 2 x 8 x 16—you get 3072, the common denominator.

    b. *Visual method.* Visually you can see that 48 is also a denominator common to all the fractions in the preceding example and is much smaller and easier to work with than 3072; 48 is also the *lowest* common denominator. Obtaining the LCD by the visual method is not always easy. The best starting point is to try the denominator which is largest; if it does not work, double it. If doubling the largest denominator does not work, triple it; eventually you will arrive at a common denominator. You must always change the denominators to their LCD before adding, subtracting, or comparing fractions.

    c. *Expressing fractions in terms of the LCD.* After you have established the lowest common denominator for the fractions with which you are working, you must express each fraction in terms of the LCD. This is accomplished by dividing the denominator of the fraction into the LCD and then multiplying both the numerator and denominator by the resulting number. After this has been done for all the fractions involved, you may proceed to add, subtract, or compare.

  17. **Adding fractions.** In the preceding paragraphs we have defined fractions, stated the rules applying to fractions, and given you the necessary information to work with fractions. Now you will work with examples which have been broken down in step procedures to show how this information is used.

    a. *Proper fractions.*

    Example: Add $\frac{3}{4}, \frac{1}{8}$, and $\frac{5}{6}$.

● *Step 1.* Find the LCD. Visually, you find the LCD to be 24, since 4 will divide into 24, 6 times; 8 will divide into 24, 3 times; and 6 will divide into 24, 4 times.

● *Step 2.* Convert each fraction to similar terms using the LCD. $24 \div 4 = 6$; therefore, $\frac{3}{4} \times \frac{6}{6} = \frac{18}{24}$; $24 \div 8 = 3$; therefore, $\frac{1}{8} \times \frac{3}{3} = \frac{3}{24}$; $24 \div 6 = 4$; therefore, $\frac{5}{6} \times \frac{4}{4} = \frac{20}{24}$.

● *Step 3.* Add the numerators and place the resulting sum over the common denominator. Thus: $18 + 3 + 20 = 41$. Therefore, the sum is $\frac{41}{24}$, which, when reduced to lowest terms, is $1\frac{17}{24}$.

    b. *Mixed numbers and fractions.*

    Example: Find the sum of $1\frac{1}{3}, 2\frac{1}{4}$, and $\frac{1}{2}$.

● *Step 1.* When working with mixed numbers, add all the whole numbers first. $1 + 2 = 3$.

● *Step 2.* Find the LCD for the fractions. By the visual method, you arrive at the LCD as being 12. Change the fractions to common terms. $\frac{1}{3} = \frac{4}{12}$; $\frac{1}{4} = \frac{3}{12}$; $\frac{1}{2} = \frac{6}{12}$.

● *Step 3.* Add the numerator. $4 + 3 + 6 = 13$. Place the resulting number (13) over the LCD: $\frac{13}{12}$, which, reduced to lowest terms, is $1\frac{1}{12}$.

● *Step 4.* Add the $1\frac{1}{12}$ to the whole number from step 1: $1\frac{1}{12} + 3 = 4\frac{1}{12}$.

  18. **Subtracting fractions**

    a. *Basic method.* The procedure for subtracting fractions is basically the same as adding them.

    Example: Subtract $\frac{3}{4}$ from $\frac{9}{10}$.

● *Step 1.* Find the LCD. By the multiplication method you find a common denominator to be 40 (4 x 10). On visual examination, however, you see that 20 is the *lowest* common denominator.

● *Step 2.* Convert each fraction to similar terms using the LCD. Dividing the 4 into 20 you get 5, which when multiplied by the numerator (5 x 3 = 15) gives $\frac{15}{20}$. Doing the same with the $\frac{9}{10}$, 20 divided by 10 = 2; 2 x 9 = 18, therefore, $\frac{18}{20}$.

● *Step 3.* Subtract the two numerators, 18 − 15 = 3. Place this number (3) over the LCD and arrive at the answer: $\frac{3}{20}$.

    b. Subtracting larger from smaller. A problem arises in mixed numbers when the fraction portion of the number being subtracted is larger than the fraction portion of the bigger number.

    Example: Subtract $1\frac{2}{3}$ from $3\frac{1}{2}$.

● *Step 1.* Find the LCD. Visually, you see that it is 6.

● *Step 2.* Express both fractions in terms of the LCD. $3\frac{1}{2} = 3\frac{3}{6}$; $1\frac{2}{3} = 1\frac{4}{6}$.

● *Step 3.* Subtract:
$$\begin{array}{r} 3\frac{3}{6} \\ - 1\frac{4}{6} \end{array}$$

You can't take $\frac{4}{6}$ from $\frac{3}{6}$. Therefore, you will have to convert the whole number (part of it in this case) to a fraction so that you may subtract. By taking 1 from $3\frac{3}{6}$ and changing it to $\frac{6}{6}$ and adding it to the $\frac{3}{6}$ you already have, you get $2\frac{9}{6}$.

You can now subtract:
$$\begin{array}{r} 2\frac{9}{6} \\ - 1\frac{4}{6} \\ \hline 1\frac{5}{6} \end{array}$$

    c. Alternate method. An alternate method is to change *all* whole numbers to fractions before subtracting and then reduce the answer to its lowest terms.

    Example: Subtract $2\frac{1}{2}$ from $4\frac{1}{4}$.

● *Step 1.* Find the LCD visually, or by the multiplication method, and you arrive at the LCD of 4.

● *Step 2.* Express all numbers (including the whole number portions) in terms of the LCD: $2\frac{1}{2} = \frac{10}{4}$ and $4\frac{1}{4} = \frac{17}{4}$.

● *Step 3.* Subtract:
$$\begin{array}{r} \frac{17}{4} \\ - \frac{10}{4} \\ \hline \frac{7}{4} \end{array}$$

● *Step 4.* Reduce to lowest terms: $\frac{7}{4} = 1\frac{3}{4}$, answer.

19. Multiplying fractions. Going back to the three general rules, you know that multiplying the numerator or dividing the denominator by a given number, multiplies the value of the fraction by that number.

    a. Multiplying fractions by multiplying the numerator.

    Example: Applying the rule, multiply $\frac{3}{4}$ by 8.

● *Step 1.* Multiply the numerator: 3 x 8 = 24. Place the resulting number (24) over original denominator: $\frac{24}{4}$

● *Step 2.* Reduce to lowest terms: $\frac{24}{4} = \frac{6}{1} = 6$, answer.

    b. Multiplying fractions by dividing the denominator.

    Example: Applying the rule, multiply $\frac{3}{4}$ by 2.

● *Step 1.* Divide the denominator: 4 ÷ 2 = 2. Placing the original numerator (3) over the new denominator, you have $\frac{3}{2}$.

● *Step 2.* Reduce to lowest terms: $\frac{3}{2} = 1\frac{1}{2}$, answer.

c. *Multiplying fractions by fractions.* To multiply two or more fractions, multiply the numerators and denominators separately and reduce the obtained fraction to lowest terms.

Example: Multiply $\frac{7}{9}$ by $\frac{6}{14}$.

● *Step 1.* Multiply the numerators: 7 x 6 = 42, the new numerator.

● *Step 2.* Multiply the denominators: 9 x 14 = 126, the new denominator.

● *Step 3.* Make a fraction of the new numbers: $\frac{42}{126}$.

● *Step 4.* Reduce to lowest terms: $\frac{42}{126} = \frac{1}{3}$, answer.

d. *Multiplying fractions by fractions using cancellation.* Cancellation is a process of dividing both numerator and denominator of fractions by the same number. It is like reducing to lowest terms. When two or more fractions are to be multiplied (or divided), cancellation between the numerators and denominators not only works, but is time saving in most cases.

Example: Multiply the following: $\frac{7}{9} \times \frac{6}{14} \times \frac{1}{2}$.

● *Step 1.* Here you will divide seven into both numerator and denominator, making the 7 a 1 and the 14 a 2: $\frac{1}{9} \times \frac{6}{2} \times \frac{1}{2} =$

● *Step 2.* Here you will divide both the numerator and denominator by two, making the 6 a 3 and 2 a 1: $\frac{1}{9} \times \frac{3}{2} \times \frac{1}{1} =$

● *Step 3.* Here you will divide both numerator and denominator by three as before. No more such division is possible, so you multiply the numerators together and the denominators together, and if necessary, reduce to lowest terms: $\frac{1}{3} \times \frac{1}{2} \times \frac{1}{1} =$

● *Step 4.* Multiply the numerators and denominators: $\frac{1}{3} \times \frac{1}{2} \times \frac{1}{1} = \frac{1}{6}$, the answer.

In this example, you have made individual steps out of each of the division steps. In a real situation, you would do all of this in one step, as shown in the next two examples.

Example: Multiply $\frac{7}{9} \times \frac{6}{14} \times \frac{1}{2}$; $\frac{\cancel{7}}{\cancel{9}} \times \frac{\cancel{6}}{\cancel{14}} \times \frac{1}{2}$ = $\frac{1}{6}$, answer.

Example: Multiply $\frac{3}{10} \times \frac{9}{26} \times \frac{26}{54}$; $\frac{\cancel{3}}{10} \times \frac{9}{\cancel{26}} \times \frac{\cancel{26}}{\cancel{54}} = \frac{1}{20}$, answer.

e. *Multiplying two or more numbers, one or more of which is a mixed number.* To multiply mixed numbers, you must change them first to improper fractions, then proceed as with regular fractions.

Example: Multiply $\frac{1}{4} \times 1\frac{5}{8} \times 1\frac{1}{2} \times 5\frac{1}{3}$.

● *Step 1.* Change all mixed numbers to improper fractions: $\frac{1}{4} \times \frac{13}{8} \times \frac{3}{2} \times \frac{16}{3}$

● *Step 2.* Cancel and reduce to lowest terms:

$\frac{1}{4} \times \frac{13}{\cancel{8}} \times \frac{\cancel{3}}{\cancel{2}} \times \frac{\cancel{16}}{\cancel{3}} = \frac{13}{4} = 3\frac{1}{4}$.

20. Dividing fractions

a. Again going back to the three general rules, "If the numerator is divided or the denominator multiplied by a given number, the value of the fraction is divided by that number," you have the basis for division among fractions. In order to avoid error, it is best to put a 1 over the whole number, so that you do not inadvertently multiply the numerator instead of the denominator.

Example: Divide $\frac{3}{4}$ by 3. Multiply the denominator of the fraction by 3: $\frac{3}{4} \times \frac{1}{3} = \frac{3}{12} = \frac{1}{4}$.

   b. To divide a whole number or a fraction by a fraction, *invert* the divisor (the number by which you are dividing). This has the effect of placing a 1 over the fraction. Thus, inverting $\frac{2}{3}$ gives us $\frac{3}{2}$, or: $\frac{1}{\frac{2}{3}} = \frac{\frac{3}{3}}{\frac{2}{3}} = \frac{3}{2}$.

   (1) Example: Divide 4 by $\frac{1}{3}$. Invert the fraction by which you are dividing: $4 \times \frac{3}{1} = \frac{12}{1} = 12$.

   (2) Example: Divide $\frac{1}{4}$ by $\frac{1}{8}$. Invert the $\frac{1}{8}$; $\frac{1}{4} \times \frac{\cancel{8}^{2}}{1} = 2$.

   (3) Example: Divide $2\frac{1}{2}$ by $1\frac{1}{4}$. Here you must first change the mixed numbers to improper fractions, then proceed as before.

$2\frac{1}{2} = \frac{5}{2}; 1\frac{1}{4} = \frac{5}{4}.$

$\frac{5}{2} \div \frac{5}{4} = \frac{\cancel{5}^{1}}{\cancel{2}_{1}} \times \frac{\cancel{4}^{2}}{\cancel{5}_{1}} = \frac{2}{1} = 2.$

21. Decimals

   a. Writing decimals. Fractions that have 10 or any power of 10 for denominators are called decimal fractions. *For example,* $\frac{1}{10}$, $\frac{3}{100}$, $\frac{126}{1000}$, and $\frac{1234}{10000}$ are decimal fractions. In writing decimals, the denominators can be omitted and a decimal point (.) placed in the numerator to show what the denominator is. There are as many digits *after* the decimal point as there were zeros in the denominator. Taking the examples above—

$\frac{1}{10} = 0.1$, $\frac{3}{100} = 0.03$, $\frac{126}{1000} = 0.126$, $\frac{1234}{10000} = 0.1234$.

Where there are less digits in the numerator than there are zeros in the denominator, zeros must be placed between the decimal point and the numerator as in $\frac{25}{10,000} = 0.0025$, and $\frac{21}{100,000} = 0.00021$. Be very careful to place the zeros to the right of the decimal and before (to the left of) the numerator.

   b. Movement of decimal point. Any error in the placement of the decimal is serious, for each movement of the decimal point to the right or left produces an error of tenfold. To illustrate what happens, consider the difference between $1.00, $10.00, $100.00, and $1,000.00. In each case, the decimal has been moved one place to the right and in each case, the amount of money represented has been multiplied ten times. Similarly, the dose of nitroglycerin is 0.4 mg.; to give a patient 4.0 mg. is a serious error. For this reason, be extremely cautious and exact when working with decimals.

22. Adding decimals

   a. When adding decimals, *always* make sure the decimal points are directly under each other. The actual addition is then the same as with whole numbers.

   b. The following three examples demonstrate the necessity of having the decimal points in line under each other. Compare examples (1) and (2) with example (3).

   (1) Example: Add $100.25, $50.69, and $18.10.

$$\begin{array}{r} \$100.25 \\ 50.69 \\ 18.10 \\ \hline \$169.04 \end{array}$$

   (2) Example: Add 21.25, 36.17, 18.19, and 7.03.

$$\begin{array}{r} 21.25 \\ 36.17 \\ 18.19 \\ 7.03 \\ \hline 82.64 \end{array}$$

(3) Example: Add 1.324, 2347.1, 0.68235, and 11.0001. Remember to line up the decimal points!

```
   1.324
2347.1
   0.68235
  11.0001
─────────
2360.10645
```

23. Subtracting decimals

a. Again the decimal points must be placed directly beneath each other, and again the procedure is the same as with whole numbers.

b. The following two examples also demonstrate the necessity of having the decimal points in line. Study example (2) carefully. Here we must add zeros at the end of the shorter numbers so that we have something to subtract from. Adding zeros at the right of the number after the decimal point has no effect on the value of the number. Zeros cannot, however, be added before the number after a decimal point, or after a number before a decimal point.

(1) Example: Subtract 11.59 from 102.21.

```
102.21
 11.59
──────
 90.62
```

(2) Example: Subtract .675061 from 2.31.

```
2.310000
 .675061
────────
1.634939
```

Thus, 2.31 is the same as 2.310000. But 2.31 is NOT equal to 2.0031 or 20.31.

24. Multiplication of decimals.
The basic principle in multiplication of decimals is that the number of places to the right of the decimal point in the product (answer) is the *sum* of the decimal points in the factors (numbers being multiplied).

Example: 43.789 (3 places to right of decimal)
× .02 (2 places to right of decimal)

Product: .87578 (3 + 2 = 5 places to right of decimal)

25. Division of decimals

a. How would you go about determining how much of a powder to pack into each of 12 capsules to evenly divide 64.8 grains of medication? You would divide 64.8 by 12. This division is shown below.

```
        5.4
    ──────
12 / 64.8
     60
     ──
      4 8
      4 8
```

b. Above you have divided and placed a decimal one place from the right because there was one place in the amount of powder. Division of a decimal by another decimal is basically the same except for one modification. We know that multiplying the numerator and the denominator each by the same number has no effect on the fraction. For this reason, we can eliminate the decimal from the divisor.

(1) Example: Divide 225.6648 by 0.8.

● *Step 1.* Multiply both the numbers by 10 (simply moving the decimal one place to the right in each case): $08 \overline{)2256.648}$.

● *Step 2.* Now the decimal will be correctly situated simply by placing it directly above the other decimal.

```
        282.081
    ──────────
08 / 2256.648
     16
     ──
      65
      64
      ──
       16
       16
       ──
        064
        064
        ───
         08
         08
```

(2) Example: Divide 1.23456 by 0.02.

$0.02 \overline{)1.23456}$

● *Step 1.* Multiply both numbers by 100 (simply moving the decimal two places to the right in each case).

$002 \overline{)123.456}$

● *Step 2.* Now the decimal will be correctly situated simply by placing it directly above the other decimal.

$$\begin{array}{r}61.728\\002\overline{)123.456}\\\underline{12}\\03\\\underline{02}\\14\\\underline{14}\\05\\\underline{04}\\16\\\underline{16}\end{array}$$

26. Roman numerals. Roman numerals are used in writing prescriptions. They are used to specify the amounts of ingredients when the apothecary system is being used, for example, "Codeine Sulfate gr. iii." They are used to specify the number of units (capsules, tablets, powders, or suppositories) to be dispensed, for example, "Disp. xxiv." And, lastly, they are used in the signa or directions to the patient, for example, "tabs. ii stat, then i q iv h." You should therefore be thoroughly familiar with the system of Roman numerals used in pharmacy. The basic symbols or numerals are—

ss or $\overline{ss}$	1/2
i	1
v	5
x	10
L	50
C	100
D	500
M	1000

These basic numerals may be combined to represent *any* number and there are definite rules for the manner in which they are combined. The rules for Roman numerals are as follows:

a. Fractions. Except for "ss" meaning one-half (1/2), all other fractions are represented by the Arabic numeral, for example, 1/4, 3/8, 1/120.

b. Repeating numerals. Numerals may be repeated and when they are, the value of the number is repeated. Thus iii or III is 3, xxx is 30, and ccc is 300. Any numeral that would be the same as another when repeated is NOT repeated. *For example*, vv is NOT used for 10 (5 + 5) because x is 10. LL is NOT used for 100 (C = 100).

c. Smaller numerals before larger. A smaller numeral placed before a larger one is subtracted from that numeral. Only one number can be subtracted in this way. Thus iv (5 − 1) = 4, ix (10 − 1) = 9; XC (100 − 10) = 90; etc. But 3 is *never* written iiv.

d. Smaller numerals after larger. A smaller numeral placed after a larger one is added to it as viii = (5 + 3) = 8; xiii (10 + 3) = 13; CLX = (100 + 50 + 10) = 160.

e. Smaller numeral between two larger. A smaller numeral between two larger ones is ALWAYS subtracted from the larger numeral which follows it as CXL (100 + (50 − 10)) = 140; MCMLXV (1000 + (1000 − 100) + 50 + 10 + 5) = 1965.

f. Dotting the one. A dot over the numeral representing 1(i) is often used to distinguish it from a portion of the numeral v. When poorly written, \ / and v may be very similar. If the ones are dotted however, \ / can never be mistaken for 5. As a further precaution against error, the last i may be replaced by a j; 3 written in this manner would be written iij.

g. Table of Roman numerals. Table 2-1 shows Roman numerals and their equivalents. Memorize this chart. You must know these numerals as well as you do Arabic numerals.

Table 1. The Roman Numerals

ss	=	½	x	=	10	xx	=	20	li	=	51
i	=	1	xi	=	11	xxi	=	21	lix	=	59
ii	=	2	xii	=	12	xxix	=	29	lx	=	60
iii	=	3	xiii	=	13	xxx	=	30	lxx	=	70
iv	=	4	xiv	=	14	xxxi	=	31	lxxx	=	80
v	=	5	xv	=	15	xxxix	=	39	xc	=	90
vi	=	6	xvi	=	16	xl	=	40	c	=	100
vii	=	7	xvii	=	17	xli	=	41	ci	=	101
viii	=	8	xviii	=	18	xlix	=	49	cxxi	=	121
ix	=	9	xix	=	19	l	=	50	d	=	500
									m	=	1000

27. Weights and measures. Metrology is the study of measurement as applied to length, weight, and volume. During your study of pharmacy in your Army career, you will constantly be dealing with it, weighing, measuring, or transposing. To be effective, both while you are learning and while you are practicing pharmacy, you must have certain tables and equivalents *committed to memory*. The time you spend memorizing the tables of weights and measures now will be repaid with interest a hundredfold. Although there are other systems of weight and measure, there are three with which the pharmacist comes into daily contact; the metric system, apothecary system, and avoirdupois system.

28. **Metric system.** The metric system of weights and measures is the legal standard in the United States. All other systems are referred to it for official comparisons. It is used as the scientific system of measuring, the world over.

   a. Units of length, weight, and volume.

   (1) Meter. The standard unit of length, the meter, may be defined as a multiple (1,650,763.73) of the wave length of the light produced by a gas-discharge lamp filled with Krypton 86. This standard permits measurements to an error of 1 part in 10 million. This extreme accuracy degree is necessary in today's missile programs.

   (2) Liter. The unit of volume in the metric system, the liter, is the volume occupied by a kilogram of water at its greatest density (4° C.), and weighed in a vacuum.

   (3) Gram. The unit of weight, the gram, is the weight of one cubic centimeter of water at its greatest density (4° C.), and weighed in a vacuum.

   NOTE
   The internationally recognized symbol for a Gram is "g." This is also the symbol used by *The United States Pharmacopeia,* XVIII, and *The National Formulary,* XIII, which were published in 1970. Previously the official abbreviation for the Gram was "Gm." This was to distinguish the Gram from the grain (gr). Another commonly used abbreviation for the Gram is "gm." The change from the abbreviation "Gm" to "g." for Gram took place while this TM was being revised. The change came too late to convert all the "Gm" abbreviations in this text to "g." As a result, Gram is still abbreviated Gm. throughout even though the accepted abbreviation is "g."

   b. Advantages of the metric system. There are several definite advantages of the metric system over the other systems—
   (1) It has universal use.

   (2) Every weight and measure has a simple relation to the meter.
   (3) Every unit is multiplied or divided by 10 to reach the next higher or lower unit. As in our system of money, it is a system of decimal progression.

   10 mills = 1 cent
   10 cents = 1 dime
   10 dimes = 1 dollar

   (4) It is the only system of weights and measures having a common standard where a unit of weight equals a unit of volume. The common standard is water. Therefore, under the standard conditions of temperature and pressure, 10 ml. of H_2O equals 10 Gm.: 100 ml. of H_2O weighs 100 Gm.

   c. Subdivisions and multiples. Each table of the metric system has a definite unit around which the subdivision and multiples are based; the meter for length, the liter for volume, and the gram for weight. Subdivisions and multiples of these principal units are indicated respectively by Latin and Greek prefixes.

   (1) Subdivisions (from Latin).

   $$\frac{1}{1000} = \text{milli}$$

   $$\frac{1}{100} = \text{centi}$$

   $$\frac{1}{10} = \text{deci}$$

   (2) Multiples (from Greek).
   10 times = Deka
   100 times = Hecto
   1000 times = Kilo

   d. Learning the metric system. When you have learned the subdivisions and multiples above, the metric system will not be difficult for you to understand or to learn. Remember that it works just like our money system. Using tables 2-2, 2-3, and 2-4, those of lengths, weights, and liquid measure, memorize the metric system.

   e. Metric weights set. Figure 2-5 depicts the standard weight set you will be using in the pharmacy. It consists of weights from 10 milligrams to 100 grams. By combining these weights, it is possible to weight substances between 10 mg. and 201 Gm. *For example,* to weigh 20.750 Gm., you would select a 20 Gm. weight, a 500 mg. weight, a 200 mg. weight, and a 50 mg. weight. The combined total of these weights is 20.750 Gm.

Table   2. Metric Table of Lengths

Lengths			Abbreviations		
10 millimeters	=	1 centimeter	10 mm.	=	1 cm
10 centimeters	=	1 decimeter	10 cm.	=	1 dm.
10 decimeters	=	1 meter	10 dm.	=	1 M.
10 Meters	=	1 Dekameter	10 M.	=	1 Dm.
10 Dekameters	=	1 Hectometer	10 Dm.	=	1 Hm.
10 Hectometers	=	1 Kilometer	10 Hm.	=	1 Km.

The metric table may also be written:

1 meter	=	1000 millimeters
	=	100 centimeters
	=	10 decimeters
	=	0.1 Dekameter
	=	0.01 Hectometer
	=	0.001 Kilometer

Table   3. Metric Table of Weights

Weights			Abbreviations		
10 milligrams	=	1 centigram	10 mg.	=	1 cg.
10 centigrams	=	1 decigram	10 cg.	=	1 dg.
10 decigrams	=	1 gram	10 dg.	=	1 Gm.
10 grams	=	1 Dekagram	10 Gm.	=	1 Dg.
10 Dekagrams	=	1 Hectogram	10 Dg.	=	1 Hg.
10 Hectograms	=	1 Kilogram	10 Hg.	=	1 Kg.

The metric table of weights may also be written:

1 gram	=	1000 milligrams
	=	100 centigrams
	=	10 decigrams
	=	0.1 Dekagram
	=	0.01 Hectogram
	=	0.001 Kilogram

Table   4. Metric Table of Liquid Measures

Liquid measures			Abbreviations		
10 milliliters	=	1 centiliter	10 ml.	=	1 cl.
10 centiliters	=	1 deciliter	10 cl.	=	1 dl.
10 deciliters	=	1 liter	10 dl.	=	1 L.
10 liters	=	1 Dekaliter	10 L.	=	1 Dl.
10 Dekaliters	=	1 Hectoliter	10 Dl.	=	1 Hl.
10 Hectoliters	=	1 Kiloliter	10 Hl.	=	1 Kl.

The metric table of liquid weights may also be written:

1 liter	=	1000 milliliters
	=	100 centiliters
	=	10 deciliters
	=	0.1 Dekaliter
	=	0.01 Hectoliter
	=	0.001 Kiloliter

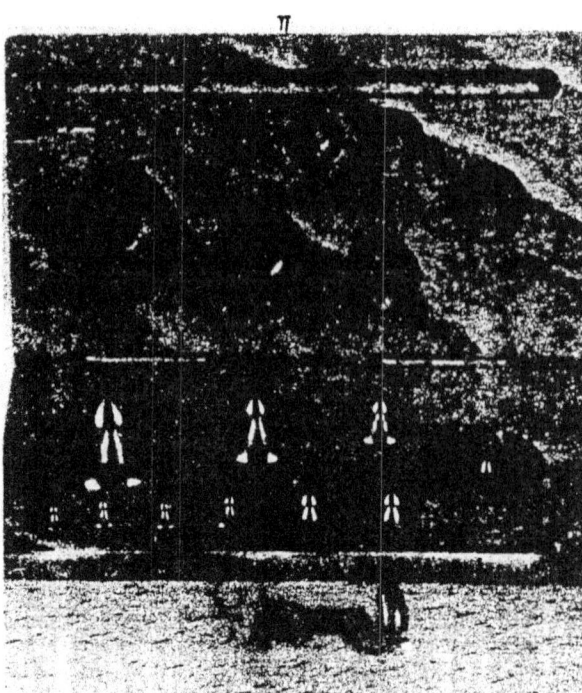

Figure   5. Metric weights.

f.   Working with the weights and measures. Now that you have reviewed decimal fractions and have learned the metric system of weights and measures, apply the two as you will be using them in your job.

(1) Example: Addition and subtraction in the metric system. Suppose you dispensed the following amounts of a powder from your stock of 4000 Gm.—28 Gm., 500 mg., 14 cg., and 2 Kg. How much powder would you have remaining?

● *Step 1.* Since you are dealing with four different denominations of weight, you cannot add or subtract until you have a common unit to work with. Since you want the answer in grams (your shelf stock having been specified in grams), it will be simplest to convert all the quantities to grams as follows:

```
  28 Gm. =    28.0  Gm.
 500 mg. =      .5  Gm.
  14 cg. =      .14 Gm.
   2 Kg. =  2000.0  Gm.
         = 2028.64  Gm. amount dispensed
```

● *Step 2.* You started with 4000 Gm. and dispensed a total of 2028.64 Gm., so by subtracting you will determine the balance on hand. Therefore:

$$4000.00 \text{ Gm.}$$
$$- 2028.64 \text{ Gm.}$$
$$1971.36 \text{ Gm. remaining}$$

NOTE

The same method is applied to liquid measure. How many ml. of alcohol would remain if you dispensed 240 from an original liter?

$$1 \text{ liter} = 1000 \text{ ml.}$$
$$- 240 \text{ ml.}$$
$$760 \text{ ml. remaining}$$

(2) Example: Multiplication. How many grams of powder would be necessary to manufacture 20 capsules, each containing 300 mg.?

$$300 \text{ mg.}$$
$$\times 20$$
$$6000 \text{ mg.} = 6.0 \text{ Gm.}$$

(3) Example: Division. How many 30 ml. bottles of cough syrup can you dispense if you have 3 liters of the syrup on hand?

$$3 \text{ liters} = 3000 \text{ ml.}$$
$$3000 \div 30 = 100 \text{ bottles, answer}$$

29. Apothecary system. Although the Army requires that all Army prescriptions be written in the metric system, the pharmacy technician must also be able to use the apothecary system. In civil practice the apothecary system is widely used and consequently many formulas are specified in terms of apothecary units. Many of the ready-made pharmaceuticals have strength and dosage listed in the apothecary system. Further, you will be filling prescriptions written by civilian prescribers who will use the apothecary system for quantity and dosage. In previous editions of the USP (Revision xiv and before), dosage of the official preparations was listed as an approximation of the apothecary system. The dosage is now completely in the metric system, the apothecary system being completely eliminated.

a. Units of weight and volume.

(1) Apothecary weight. The basic unit in the apothecary system of weight is the grain, which is approximately 64.8 mg. Divisions of the grain are expressed as fractions, for example, $\frac{1}{60}$ gr. Prescriptions will be written with a symbol for the weight denomination and a Roman numeral for the amount of that denomination. Study the table of apothecary weights and abbreviations (table 2-5). Thus, in prescriptions written in the apothecary system, you will see the following written:

Ωiii   ʒii   gr iiiss   ℥viii

Table 5. Apothecary Weights and Abbreviations

Apothecary weights			Abbreviations
20 grains	= 1 scruple		gr. xx = Ωi
3 scruples	= 1 drachm	= 60 grains	Ω iii = ʒi
8 drachms	= 1 ounce	= 480 grains	ʒviii = ℥i
12 ounces	= 1 pound	= 5760 grains	℥xii = 1 lb.

(2) Apothecary liquid measure. The basic unit of the apothecary system of fluid measure is the minim (♏). Study the table of apothecary liquid measure below in table 2-6. Prescriptions are written with a symbol for the denomination to be used. Thus in prescriptions written in the apothecary system for liquids, you will see quantities such as the following:

f ℥ ss   f ʒ ¼   ♏xii   f ℥ viii

(3) Apothecary weights. Apothecary weights used in pharmacy are of two types—cylindrical weights and coin weights.

(a) Apothecary cylindrical weights. The apothecary cylindrical weights are

Table 6. Apothecary Fluid Measure and Abbreviations

Apothecary fluid measure			Abbreviation	
60 minims	= 1 fluidrachm	=	♏lx	= f ʒi
8 fluidrachm	= 1 fluidounce	= 480 minims	f ʒviii	= f ℥i
16 fluidounce	= 1 pint	= 7,680 minims	f ℥vxi	= Oi
2 pints	= 1 quart	= 32 fluidounces	Oii	= qt i
4 quarts	= 1 gallon	= 128 fluidounces	qt iv	= Ci

similar to the metric weights depicted in figure 2-5. They usually range from one-half scruple to two drachms. The set contains grain weights in the form of wires; the number of sides indicates the number of grains (fig. 2-6).

   (b) *Apothecary coin weights.* Coin-type weights which have the weight embossed on their surfaces are particularly subject to error and should not be used.

   b. *Converting between denominations.* It is often convenient to express a weight or measure in its equivalent in a lower or higher denomination. This can be easily accomplished by either multiplying or dividing the weight by the number of units that equals either the higher or lower measure.

   (1) *Example:* Express 3/4 quart in its lowest terms in the apothecary system.

● *Step 1.* Since 2 pints = 1 quart; 2 x 3/4 = 1 1/2 pints which can be expressed—pt ii x qt 3/4 = pt iss.

● *Step 2.* Put aside and save the whole number, the one pint, and break the fraction to its next lowest terms.
$$1 \text{ pint} = 16 \text{ fluidounces}$$
$$\text{so, } 16 \text{ fluidounces} \times 1/2 = 8 \text{ fluidounces}$$
$$\text{or, } f\!\!\!\!3 \text{ xvi} \times \text{pt ss} = f\!\!\!\!3 \text{ viii}$$

● *Step 3.* Continue in this manner, changing each remaining fraction to the next lower denomination. In this case, however, you need go no further, 8 ounces is even. Now you have the whole pint saved from step 2, which equals 16 ounces plus the 8 ounces from step 3, or a total of 24 fluidounces for the answer.

   (2) *Example:* Express 2/5 gallon in its lowest apothecary terms.

● *Step 1.* 1 gallon = 8 pints.
$$8 \times 2/5 = 3\ 1/5 \text{ pt}$$
$$\text{or, pt viii} = \text{gal i}$$
$$\text{pt viii} \times \text{gal } 2/5 = \text{pt iii } 1/5$$

● *Step 2.* Continue in this manner, saving the whole and breaking the fraction to its next lowest terms:
$$fl\!\!\!\!3 \text{ xvi} \times \text{pt } 1/5 = f\!\!\!\!3 \text{ iii } 1/5$$
$$fl\!\!\!\!3 \text{ xviii} \times fl\!\!\!\!3\ 1/5 = fl\!\!\!\!3 \text{ i } 3/5$$
$$\mathfrak{m} \text{lx} \times fl\!\!\!\!3\ 3/5 = \mathfrak{m} \text{xxxvi}$$

● *Step 3.* Putting the numbers previously saved together in sequence, you arrive at the answer: 2/5 gallons = 3 pints, 3 fluidounces, 1 fluidrachm, and 36 minims; or gallon 2/5 = ℥iii, fl ℥ iii, fl ℨ i, ♏ xxxvi.

   (3) *Example:* In order to proceed from a lower measure to highest terms, the procedure is just opposite. Divide the measure by the number of units of that measure that equals one unit of the next higher measure. Express 57,688 minims in its highest terms.

● *Step 1.* 60 minims = 1 fluidrachm, therefore

```
         961 ────→ 961 fl ℨ
    60/57688
         540
         ───
         368
         360
         ───
          88
          60
          ──
          28 ────→ 28 minims
```
Save the minims left over and break down the fluidrachms.

● *Step 2.* 8 fluidrachms = 1 fluidounce, therefore

```
         120 ────→ 120 fl ℨ
      8/961
         8
         ──
         16
         16
         ──
         01
          0
         ──
          1 ────→ 1 fluid ℨ
```
Save the fluidrachms and break down the fluidounces.

● *Step 3.* 16 fluidounces = 1 pint, therefore

```
           7 ────→ 7 pints
     16/120
        112
        ───
          8 ────→ 8 fluidounces
```
Save the fluidounces and change the pints to the next higher value (quarts).

● *Step 4.* 2 fluid pints = 1 fluid quart, therefore

```
           3 ────→ 3 quarts
       2/7
         6
         ──
         1 ────→ 1 pint
```

● *Step 5.* Now, combine the various quantities you have saved in previous steps. Your answer is:

57,688 minims = 3 qts, 1 pt, 8 f℥ , 1 f𝔇 , 28 minims.

(4) Checking your answers. You can check your answers in both procedures by just reversing the procedure.

● In example (2), you converted 2/5 gallon to 3 pints, 3 fluidounces, 1 fluidrachm, and 36 minims. Going in reverse to check the accuracy:

60 minims = 1 fluidrachm

$\frac{36}{60}$ minims = 3/5 fluidrachm

3/5 + 1 = 1 3/5 fluidrachms
8 fluidrachms = 1 fluidounce
1 3/5 fluidrachms = 1/5 fluidounce
1/5 + 3 = 3 1/5 fluidounces
16 fluidounces = 1 pint
3 1/5 fluidounces = 1/5 pint
1/5 + 3 = 3 1/5 pints
8 pints = 1 gallon
3 1/5 pints = 2/5 gallon—the answer checks.

● In example (3), you converted 57,688 minims to 7 pints, 8 fluidounces, 1 fluidrachm, and 28 minims. To check this answer, you again proceed in reverse.

7 pt, 8 fl℥, 1 fl𝔇 + 28 minims ⟶ 28 minims
7 pt, 8 fl℥, 1 fl𝔇
1 fl𝔇 = 60 minims ⟶ 60 minims
7 pt, 8 fl℥
8 fl℥ = 64 fl𝔇 (8 x 8)
64 fl𝔇 = ⟶ 3,840 minims
(64 x 60)
7 pt = 112 fl℥ = 896 fl𝔇 = ⟶ 53,760 minims
(112 x 8) (896 x 60)
adding the columns of minims ⟶ 57,688 minims
our answer checks.

c. Addition and subtraction. The arithmetic involved in the apothecary system is slightly more involved than that of the metric system. In the metric system, the units increase by multiples of ten. However, the apothecary system has no uniform scale of variation. You are again confronted with the problem that quantities of like denomination must be added or subtracted first, then converted to lowest terms. To illustrate this, look at the following addition problem.

(1) Example:
4 lb, 3 ℥ , 4 𝔇 , 1 𝔈 , 18 gr.
+ 8 lb, 2 ℥ , 3 𝔇 , 2 𝔈 , 19 gr.

● *Step 1.* By simple addition, adding pounds to pounds, ounces to ounces, you get—
4 lb, 3 ℥ , 4 𝔇 , 1 𝔈 , 18 gr.
+ 8 lb, 2 ℥ , 3 𝔇 , 2 𝔈 , 19 gr.
12 lb, 5 ℥ , 7 𝔇 , 3 𝔈 , 37 gr.

● *Step 2.* This answer is not in its reduced terms, because 37 grains equals one scruple plus 17 grains, 3 scruples equal a drachm, and so on. To reduce this answer, begin at the right and work to the left, changing each quantity possible to the next higher denomination. Twenty grains equals one scruple, leaving 17 grains and adding 1 scruple to the 3 previously in the column. Likewise, since there are 3 scruples to the drachm, you must convert 3 of the 4 scruples you now have in this column to 1 drachm, leaving 1 𝔈 and increasing the drachms to 8. There being 8 drachms to the ounce, you have no drachms remaining, but increase the ounces to 6. The final reduced answer then beomes 12 lb, 6 ℥ , 1 𝔈 , 17 gr.

(2) Example: Subtract 4 lb, 6 ℥ , 4 𝔇 , 1 𝔈 , 19 gr. from 6 lb, 8 ℥ , 5 𝔇 , 2 𝔈 , 15 gr.

● *Step 1.* Set up for subtraction.
6 lb, 8 ℥ , 5 𝔇 , 2 𝔈 , 15 gr.
− 4 lb, 6 ℥ , 4 𝔇 , 1 𝔈 , 19 gr.

Since you could not take 19 grains from 15 grains, it is necessary to convert one scruple to grains, reducing the number of scruples in the upper figure to 1 and increasing the grains to 35. You may never have a negative number in subtracting weights and measures.

● *Step 2.* Having converted the scruple to grains, your problem becomes:
6 lb, 8 ℥ , 5 𝔇 , 1 𝔈 , 35 gr.
− 4 lb, 6 ℥ , 4 𝔇 , 1 𝔈 , 19 gr.
2 lb, 2 ℥ , 1 𝔇 , 0 𝔈 , 16 gr.

d. Multiplication and division.
(1) Example: Multiplication. Multiplication of compound numbers such as arise in the apothecary system may be accomplished in several ways, the easiest of which is to multiply each denomination individually, then reduce the answer. Multiply 2 gal, 3 qt, 1 pt, 9 f℥ , 7 f𝔇 , 18 min. by 6.

● *Step 1.*
2 gal, 3 qt, 1 pt, 9 f℥ , 7 f𝔇 , 81 min.
x 6
12 gal, 18 qt, 6 pt, 54 f℥ , 42 f𝔇 , 108 min.

19

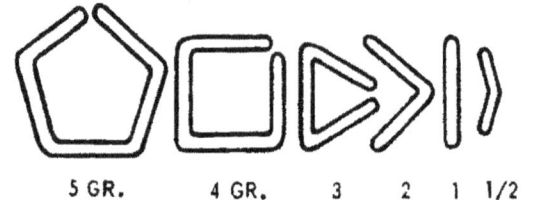

Figure 6. Apothecary grain weights.

Table 7. Approximate Equivalents

Weight					
Metric	Approx apothecary	Metric	Approx apothecary	Metric	Approx apothecary
0.1 mg.	1/600 gr.	6 mg.	1/10 gr.	0.1 Gm.	1-1/2 gr.
0.2 mg.	1/300 gr.	8 mg.	1/8 gr.	0.12 Gm.	2 gr.
0.3 mg.	1/200 gr.	10 mg.	1/6 gr.	0.15 Gm.	2-1/2 gr.
0.4 mg.	1/150 gr.	12 mg.	1/5 gr.	0.2 Gm.	3 gr.
0.5 mg.	1/120 gr.	15 mg.	1/4 gr.	0.3 Gm.	5 gr.
0.6 mg.	1/100 gr.	20 mg.	1/3 gr.	0.5 Gm.	7-1/2 gr.
1 mg.	1/60 gr.	25 mg.	3/8 gr.	0.6 Gm.	10 gr.
1.2 mg.	1/50 gr.	30 mg.	1/2 gr.	1 Gm.	15 gr.
2 mg.	1/30 gr.	50 mg.	3/4 gr.	1.5 Gm.	22 gr.
3 mg.	1/20 gr.	60 mg.	1 gr.	2 Gm.	30 gr.
4 mg.	1/15 gr.	75 mg.	1-1/4 gr.	3 Gm.	45 gr.
5 mg.	1/12 gr.	90 mg.	1-1/2 gr.	4 Gm.	60 gr. (1 drachm)
				5 Gm.	75 gr.
				7.5 Gm.	2 drachms
				15 Gm.	4 drachms
				30 Gm.	1 ounce
Liquid Measure					
Metric	Approx apothecary	Metric	Approx apothecary	Metric	Approx apothecary
0.03 ml.	1/2 minim	0.6 ml.	10 minims	15 ml.	4 f. drachms (1/2 oz)
0.05 ml.	3/4 minim	0.75 ml.	12 minims	30 ml.	1 f. ounce
0.06 ml.	1 minim	1 ml.	15 minims	60 ml.	2 f. ounces
0.1 ml.	1-1/2 minims	2 ml.	30 minims	120 ml.	4 f. ounces
0.2 ml.	3 minims	3 ml.	45 minims	250 ml.	8 f. ounces
0.25 ml.	4 minims	4 ml.	60 minims	500 ml.	16 f. ounces (1 pint)
0.3 ml.	5 minims	5 ml.	1 f. drachm	1000 ml.	1 quart
0.5 ml.	8 minims	10 ml.	2 f. drachms		

N.B. These are *approximate* equivalents. They may be used to compare prepared dosage forms such as tablets, capsules, and solutions. For converting *specific* quantities as are called for in formulas, use the exact equivalents provided in the U.S.P. For prescription compounding, use the exact equivalents rounded to 3 significant figures.

Step 2. Simply reduce the above answer to the lowest terms as previously explained.

17 gal, 2 qt, 1 pt, 11 f℥, 3 fℨ, 48 min.

(2) Example: Division (usual method). Division of compound numbers is best done by dividing the highest measure first, keeping the whole number obtained and converting any remainder to the next smaller denomination and adding it to the given quantity. Then continue the division. Divide 8 gal, 2 qt, 1 pt by 3.

- *Step 1.*
  8 gal ÷ 3 = 2 gal (+ 2 gal remainder)
  2 gal = 8 qt + original 2 qt = 10 qt.

- *Step 2.*
  10 qt ÷ 3 = 3 qt (+ 1 qt remainder)
  1 qt = 2 pt + original 1 pt + 3 pt.

- *Step 3.*
  3 pt ÷ 3 = 1 pt.

- *Step 4.* Add the products from all steps (not the remainders!).
  2 gal, 3 qt, 1 pt, answer.

(3) Example: Division (alternate method). An alternate method is to convert the amounts to their lowest form; in this case, pints, then convert back to highest terms after dividing. Divide 8 gal, 2 qt, 1 pt by 3.

- *Step 1.*
  8 gal = 64 pt
  2 qt = 4 pt
  1 pt = 1 pt
  total = 69 pt

- *Step 2.* Divide.
  69 ÷ 3 = 23 pt

- *Step 3.* Convert back to highest terms.
  23 pt = 11 qt, 1 pt
  11 qt = 2 gal, 3 qt
  2 gal, 3 qt, 1 pt, answer.

30. Avoirdupois system. In the United States all items sold by weight are commercially bought and sold by avoirdupois weight. Exceptions to this rule include gems and precious metals. The weight which appears on a scale when you weigh yourself is avoirdupois weight. Unless expressly stated, all drugs and chemicals are bought and sold by avoirdupois weight. Therefore, it is *extremely* important to note that in receiving narcotics from the warehouse, an ounce bottle contains 437.5 grains (avoirdupois ounce), not 480 grains (apothecary ounce). As you can readily see, serious error could result in your narcotic records if you did not understand this principle. The grain is common to BOTH the avoirdupois and the apothecary system, *but* the ounces and pounds are different. Study the comparison below.

Apothecary ounce = 480.0 grains
Avoirdupois ounce = 437.5 grains
            = 42.5 grains *difference*

Apothecary pound = 12 oz x 480 grains = 5760 grains
Avoirdupois pound = 16 oz x 437.5 grains = 7000 grains
                                           1240 grains *difference*

31. Relationship and approximate equivalents. The metric system, apothecary system, and avoirdupois system are all used extensively by the pharmacy technician. Because you have and use three separate systems of weight and measure, it is necessary to understand their relationship and know how to convert from one to the other quickly and accurately.

   a. Some relationships to remember.
- *Remember:* The pharmacist receives drugs and chemicals by avoirdupois weight at 437.5 grains per ounce, 16 ounces per pound.
- *Remember:* The pharmacist dispenses prescriptions in the metric or apothecary system. The apothecary system has 480 grains per ounce and only 12 ounces per pound.
- *Remember:* One apothecary fluidounce (H_2O) weighs 454.6 grains at 25° C. There are 480 minims in an apothecary fluidounce. It follows, then, that 1 minim of water at 25° C. weighs $\frac{454.6}{480}$ = 0.95 grains.

   b. Approximate equivalents. Table 2-7 should be thoroughly memorized. These equivalents will allow conversion between systems with a *relative degree of accuracy*. A facsimile of this table should be conspicuously placed near the work area in your pharmacy as a reference and check.

c. *Exact conversion.* Exact accuracy in conversion from one system to another as is needed for compounding prescriptions cannot be accomplished using approximate equivalents. Nearly exact conversion equivalents are given in a table in the USP.

32. **Ratio and proportion**

   a. *Ratio.* Ratio is an expression of the relationship of one thing to another. For the purpose of arithmetic, ratio is the relation showing the amount by which one thing is different from another. Thus, if you have a solution of 9 grams of sodium chloride in 1000 grams of water, the ratio of NaCl to water is 9:1000 or $\frac{9}{1000}$, and is read "9 to 1000." The value of a ratio is the number obtained by dividing the first term (antecedent) by the second term (consequent); therefore, the value of 12:4 is 3.

   (1) Ratios remain constant. Multiplying or dividing BOTH terms of a ratio does not change its value. Therefore, multiplying both terms of 10:5 by 5 gives us 50:25. In either case, the ratio is the same, 2:1. The terms of a ratio taken together are called a couplet.

   (2) Equal units. Ratio can exist only between numbers of the same unit value—as ratio of percent to percent or weight to weight—but never weight to percent. (*Exception:* In pharmacy, we often make solutions which are expressed as weight to volume.) The comparing of numbers of the same unit volume follows as certainly as apples can be compared to apples and oranges to oranges, but never oranges to apples.

   (3) Examples of ratio problems:
   - What is the value of the ratio 10:100? Divide the first term by the second to get 1/10.
   - Simplify 6:36. Divide both terms by 6 to get 1:6.
   - What is the ratio between 18 percent and 9 grams? No ratio! Percent cannot be compared to grams.
   - What do the following three ratios have in common? 1:5, 3:15, 5:25. When simplified, each is 1:5 or 1/5.

   b. *Proportion.* 15:3 :: 10:2 is a proportion. It is read "15 is to 3 as 10 is to 2." Proportion is a means of showing equality between ratios. $15 \div 3 = 5$ and $10 \div 2 = 5$; they have the same value. The first and fourth terms of a proportion are called the *extremes* and the second and third terms are called the *means*. In the example cited above, 15 and 2 are the extremes; 3 and 10 are the means. The product of the extremes (15 x 2) equals the product of the means (3 x 10).

   (1) Example: 50:10 :: 25:5
   $50 \times 5 = 250;$
   $10 \times 25 = 250.$

Thus, it is apparent that if one of the numbers were an unknown, it could easily be determined as follows:

   (2) Example: If it takes 50 grains of powder to make 5 capsules, how many grains are necessary to make 3 capsules? This problem is nothing more than a proportion in which one of the terms is an unknown.

   50:x :: 5:3
   5x = 150 (arrived at by multiplying the means and extremes)
   x = 30 grains, answer (to make 3 capsules)

It is customary to let x or y represent the unknown number in proportions. Thus you find that 30 grains would be necessary to make 3 capsules.

   (3) Example: Rule of Words. Putting this example into a rule of words—"To find either extreme, multiply the means (2nd and 3rd numbers) and divide by the known extreme." Likewise, "To find either mean, multiply the extremes (1st and 4th numbers) and divide by the known mean." Notice how you progress from a statement of problem to a written proportion. If 500 Gm. of a salt solution contains 10 percent salt, to what weight must you evaporate the solution to make it 20 percent salt?

   - *Step 1.* Write down the facts.
     500 Gm. is 10%
     ? Gm. is 20%

- *Step 2.* Let x represent the unknown (?) quantity. Arbitrarily, let x take the fourth position.

- *Step 3.* Since we can compare only like articles, put the number with the same denomination as x in the third position.

- *Step 4.* Determine if the unknown is to be larger or smaller than the third number. In the preceding example, you are evaporating a solution and thus it will be smaller. Since the smaller follows the larger in the 3rd and 4th positions, the *same* must hold true of the 1st and 2d. Therefore, the larger number will be in first position, and the smaller in second position.

- *Step 5.* From the preceding 4 steps, you may conclude that—
  20:10 :: 500:x

- *Step 6.* Cross multiply (multiply the means and extremes).
  20 x = 5000

- *Step 7.* Solve for x.
  x = 5000 ÷ 20
  x = 250 Gm., the weight of the 20% solution, answer.

33. Percentage preparations. Many of the calculations you will be required to make in the pharmacy will be for the compounding and dispensing of percentage preparations (solutions or powders). The most important factor to keep in mind here is that *slight* errors in dilute preparations may be considered negligible, whereas even a slight error in a concentrated preparation may be serious. To firmly impress this in your mind, consider the difference between losing one quarter from your pocket containing ten quarters and losing ten quarters from another pocket containing 100 quarters. The loss in each case is 10 percent. In the first instance, 10 percent loss amounted to only 25 cents, while in the second instance the 10 percent loss amounted to $2.50. Thus, as the percentage of a solution or other preparation becomes greater, the error becomes more severe. The strength of a solution is the ratio of active ingredient to solvent and can be expressed as a percent or as a ratio.

  a. Percent solutions. The Latin "per centum" literally means "by hundreds." Ten percent, then, refers to 10 hundreds or 10 parts out of 100 parts. A 10-percent solution could be broken down as follows:
  Total volume of solution — 100% or 100 parts
  Solute (active ingredient) — 10% or 10 parts
  Solvent — 90% or 90 parts

In solutions of solids or gases in a liquid, the solid or gas being dissolved is called the solute, and the liquid is the solvent. In solution of liquids in liquids, we arbitrarily say that the liquid present in greater quantity is the solvent and the liquid of lesser quantity is the solute. Thus we say that in mixing 25 percent water and 75 percent alcohol, we obtain a solution of water in alcohol. Reversing the situation, 25 percent alcohol and 75 percent water, we would term a solution of alcohol in water.

  (1) Variable meaning of percentage. Percentage in solutions can have different meanings under different circumstances. In solution, you are dealing with solids which are weighed, and liquids which can be weighed or measured; thus, it is necessary to define the expression of percentage concentration of solutions. There are three different percentage solutions:

  (a) Percent weight in weight (w/w)—expresses the number of grams of a constituent in 100 grams of solution.

  (b) Percent weight in volume (w/v)—expresses the number of grams of a constituent in 100 ml. of solution, and is used in prescription practice regardless of whether water or another liquid is used.

  (c) Percent volume in volume (v/v)—expresses the number of milliliters of a constituent in 100 ml. of solution.

(2) Rules for percentage solutions. Unless specifically stipulated otherwise, the following rules hold true for prescriptions of percentage solutions:
- Mixtures of solids are weight in weight.
- Solids in liquids are weight in volume.
- Liquids in liquids are volume in volume.
- Gases in liquids are weight in volume.

For example, to make a 10-percent solution, dissolve 10 Gm. of a solid or 10 ml. of a liquid in the amount of solvent necessary (qs) to make 100 ml. of finished solution. In the apothecary system, 45.6 grains of a solid or 48 minims of a liquid dissolved in enough solvent to make 1 fluidounce would yield a 10-percent solution. Slight changes in volume attributable to changes in room temperature are negligible and may be disregarded.

  b. Percent weight in volume solutions. Weight in volume (w/v) percentage may be called the "key" to percentage and ratio solutions. You are dissolving a weight of solid in a volume of liquid (water, unless otherwise specified).

  (1) Metric system rule. Multiply the specified percentage, expressed as a decimal fraction, times the required number of ml. The resulting number will represent the number of grams of solid in the solution, or percent (decimal) x ml. = grams solute.

  (2) Apothecary system rule. Multiply the percent, expressed as a whole number times 4.5457 times fluidounces of solution required. The answer you obtain will be the number of grains of solute to be used. The weight of 1 fluidounce of water at 25° C. is 454.57 grains. Therefore, 4.5457 grains is the amount of solute necessary to prepare a 1-percent solution of 1 ounce. Expressed as a formula, this rule becomes percent (whole number) x 4.5457 x fl oz. required = grains of solute.

  (3) Example: Prepare 300 ml. of 20-percent (w/v) solution of sodium thiosulfate. How many grams of solute are necessary? How much solvent is used?

- *Step 1.* Formula.
  % (decimal) x ml. = grams solute

- *Step 2.* Substitute.
  .20 x 300 = 60 grams of solute

- *Step 3.* Since the total solution is to be 300 ml., you add enough water to the 60 grams of solute to make the finished product measure 300 ml. If you assumed that 60 grams took up 60 ml. of volume, you could deduce that 240 ml. of liquid added to the 60 grams of solute would make 300 ml. This does not hold true. Many solids when dissolved do not take up a volume equal to their weight, so you must always add enough water to make the volume up to the required amount. This bringing up to the required volume is expressed in prescriptions as "qs ad" from the Latin, and means "add a sufficient quantity."

  (4) Example: Work this similar problem in the apothecary system. Make ℥ iv (4 fluidounces) of a 20-percent solution of sodium thiosulfate.

- *Step 1.* Formula.
  % x 4.5457 x fl. oz. = grains of solute.

- *Step 2.* Substitute.
  20 x 4.5457 x 4 = 363.6 grains = (℥ vi gr iiiss)

The prescription could have been written:
  Rx Sod. Thiosulfate grs 363.6
  Pur. Water qs ad ℥ iv.

  c. Percent volume in volume solutions. To calculate percentage of solutions of one liquid in another, multiply the desired percent, as a decimal fraction, of the active ingredient times the amount of total solution desired.

  Example: How many ml. of an active ingredient must be used to produce 480 ml. of a 3-percent solution?
  480 x .03 = 34.4 ml., answer

  d. Percent weight in weight solution. In some cases, a definite finished weight of solution is required. To find the percent of solid in the solution, multiply the total weight of the finished solution desired by the percent desired, expressed as a decimal. Written as a formula this would be—Gm. total solution x % (decimal) = Gm. of active solute. By subtracting this weight (the weight of the solute) from the weight of the total solution, the weight of the liquid required as solvent is found. This weight may be converted to volume by dividing the weight of liquid required by the specific gravity of the liquid. Specific gravity will be discussed below.

  (1) Example: How many grams of acriflavine are required to manufacture 200 Gm. of a 10-percent (w/w) solution? How much glycerin will you use as the solvent? Express the amount of glycerin in both weight and volume (Sp. Gr. glycerin = 1.25).

200 x 0.10 = 20 Gm. acriflavine
200 − 20 = 180 Gm. glycerin
180 ÷ 1.25 = 144 ml. glycerin

(2) Example: Prepare 4 fluidounces of a 10-percent (w/w) solution of acriflavine in glycerin. This problem takes on more difficulty in the apothecary system. First reduce the total weight of solution to grains.

- *Step 1.* Reduce solution to grains.
  4 fl oz x 454.6 = 1818.4 grains (total solution)

- *Step 2.* 10 % of 1818.4 = 181.84 grains of acriflavine.

- *Step 3.* 1818.4 − 181.84 = 1636.56 grains of glycerin.

- *Step 4.* 1 fl oz of water weighs 454.6 grains; therefore, 1 fluidounce of glycerin weighs 454.6 x 1.25 = 568.25 gr.

- *Step 5.* Since you need 1636.56 grains of glycerin, by dividing this by the number of grains of glycerin in a fluidounce, you will obtain the volume of glycerin required in terms of fluidounces.
  1636.56 ÷ 568.25 = 2.88 fluidounces or
  f ℥ ii   f ʒ vii   ♏ii

34. Ratio preparations. Ratio is similar to percent, the entire solution is the total, the active ingredient is a certain part of the total, and the solvent or diluent is the remainder. Ratio solutions are expressed as so much in so much; for example, 1 in 10; 1 in 100; 1 in 1000. It means exactly what it says, 1 part in a total of 10 parts, or 1 part in a total of 100 parts; it does not mean 1 part plus 10 parts to give 11 parts. It is obvious that a 1 in 10 solution, therefore, is identical to a 10 percent solution. A ratio solution is expressed by parts—so many parts in a total of so many parts; 1 part in 10 parts = 1 in 10. The number of parts of active ingredient is taken as 1, and the total parts possible is variable as in 1 in 10, 1 in 20, 1 in 100. You remember in percentage, the total mixture was always 100 and the active part was variable, as 10 percent (10/100), 20 percent (20/100), or 50 percent (50/100).

a. Weight in volume solution by ratio. The following proportion is used in making ratio solutions of the weight in volume type.

$$\frac{\text{weight of solute}}{\text{wt of given volume of solution if it were water}} :: \frac{\text{one part of solute}}{\text{No. of parts of completed solution containing 1 part of solute}}$$

(1) Example: What is the ratio strength (w/v) of a solution containing 25 Gm. of solute in 250 ml. of solution?
Substitute in the preceding formula.

$$\frac{25}{250} :: \frac{1}{x}$$

$$25x = 250$$

x = 10; ratio strength, then, is 1 in 10 (1/10)
Using this formula, any one of the four parts can be found, if the other three are known.

(2) Example: If the ratio strength (w/v) of a solution is 1:25, and it contains 50 Gm. of solute, what is the total volume of the solution? Substitute:

$$\frac{50}{x} :: \frac{1}{25}$$

x = 1250 ml., the total volume of solution.

b. Volume in volume solution by ratio. Again, a simple proportion can be used to solve this type of problem.

$$\frac{\text{vol. of ingredient}}{\text{vol. of total solution}} :: \frac{\text{parts of ingredient}}{\text{parts of whole}}$$

CAUTION

The two volumes concerned *must* be expressed in the same denomination; that is, if one is expressed in ml., the other must also be ml.

(1) Example: What amount of active ingredient must be used to produce 500 ml. of a solution (v/v) with a ratio strength of 1:20? Substitute:

$$\frac{x}{500} :: \frac{1}{20}$$

$$20x = 500$$

x = 25 ml., answer

(2) Example: What is the ratio strength of a solution which contains 5 ml. of active ingredient in a total of 250 ml.? Substitute:

$$\frac{5}{250} :: \frac{1}{x}$$

$$5x = 250$$

$$x = 50$$

strength is 1 in 50 (1:50)

c. Weight to weight solution by ratio. For w/w solutions, two proportions may be expressed;

one shows the relationship between active ingredient and the total solution, the other between ingredient and diluent.

$$\frac{\text{wt ingredient}}{\text{wt mixture}} :: \frac{\text{parts of ingredient}}{\text{parts total mixture}}$$

or

$$\frac{\text{wt ingredient}}{\text{wt diluent}} :: \frac{\text{parts of ingredient}}{\text{parts of diluent}}$$

(1) Example: What is the weight in grams of a 1:10,000 (w/w) solution containing 150 mg. of active ingredient? Substituting in first formula:

$$\frac{150}{x} = \frac{1}{10,000}$$

x = 1,500,000 mg.

x = 1500 Gm. (wt of solution)

(2) Example: If 8 Gm. of a substance is dissolved in 128 ml. of water, what is the w/w ratio strength of the solution? Substituting in second formula:

$$\frac{8}{128} :: \frac{1}{x}$$

8x = 128

x = 16

1 in 16 (1:16)

35. Specific gravity. Specific gravity, abbreviated Sp. Gr., is the relation between the weights of two substances, one of which is a standard. Determination of Sp. Gr. is accomplished under specific conditions, namely, 25° C. and normal barometric pressure. Distilled water is the standard for liquids and solids, and air for gases. Specific gravity is always expressed as a decimal; the standard substance has a Sp. Gr. of 1.000. Comparing equal volumes of glycerin and water, for example, we find that glycerin is 1-1/4 times as heavy. Since the Sp. Gr. of water is 1.000, the Sp. Gr. of glycerin is 1.250.

36. Specific gravity of liquids. There are several instruments used for determination of the specific gravity of liquids. We will discuss only two here, the pycnometer and the hydrometer.

a. Pycnometer. The pycnometer (fig. 2-7) is a specific gravity bottle. Pycnometer is derived from the Greek word pykno, meaning dense, and meter, meaning measure. It is, therefore, a device for measuring density. Any small, long-necked flask made of thin glass will serve as a pycnometer. It is preferable for simplicity of calculation that the pycnometer hold some simple unit volume of

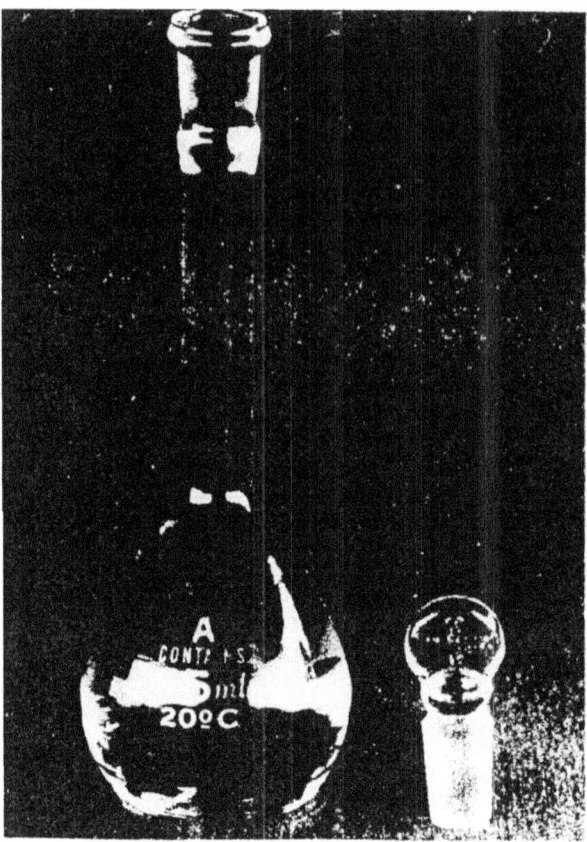

Figure 7. The pycnometer.

water, 25 Gm., 50 Gm., or 100 Gm. You will see the benefit of this in the following paragraphs. To find specific gravity using a pycnometer, proceed as follows:

(1) First, we must know the exact weight of the empty pycnometer. This is called the "tare" or "tare weight." Since dirt and moisture will affect this tare weight, it is important that the vessel be clean and dry. Make a note of the tare weight.

(2) Distilled water is then poured into the pycnometer until it reaches a convenient level in the neck. A line is marked on the pycnometer at the level of the lower edge of the meniscus (concave or convex surface of the liquid).

(3) Note the temperature of the water and record it. Now carefully weigh the pycnometer and its contents and record the combined weight.

(4) The weight of the water alone can be calculated by subtracting the tare weight of the pycnometer from the combined weight recorded in step *(3)* above. This is the weight of the water at the recorded temperature. The tare weight, temperature, and weight of the water may be permanently etched on the side of the flask for

future calculations. These figures will remain constant for all future specific gravity determinations.

(5) When the flask is again clean and dry, the specific gravity of any liquid may be taken by filling it to the same point with the liquid to be tested.

(6) Weigh the pycnometer, now containing a liquid to be tested, and subtract the tare weight of the vessel. The number resulting will be the weight of the liquid you are testing.

(7) Determine the specific gravity by substituting in this formula:

$$\text{Sp. Gr.} = \frac{\text{weight of known volume of substance}}{\text{weight of equal volume of distilled water}}$$

(8) *Example:* A pycnometer weighs 20.123 Gm. when clean and dry. When filled to a convenient level with water at 25° C., it weighs 44.678 Gm. The same bottle filled to the same level with glycerin at 25° C. weighs 50.816 Gm. What is the specific gravity of the glycerin?

- *Step 1.*

weight of glycerin + bottle =	50.816 Gm.
minus tare weight of bottle	− 20.123 Gm.
the weight of glycerin	30.693 Gm.

- *Step 2.*

weight of water + bottle =	44.678 Gm.
minus tare weight of bottle	− 20.123 Gm.
the weight of water	24.555 Gm.

- *Step 3.* Formula:

$$\text{Sp. Gr.} = \frac{\text{weight substance}}{\text{weight equal volume of water}}$$

- *Step 4.*

$$\text{Sp. Gr.} = \frac{30.693}{24.555} = 1.25 \text{ the Sp. Gr. of glycerin}$$

b. Hydrometer. The hydrometer is an instrument which gives us a quick but not as accurate a determination of specific gravity as the pycnometer. It can also be used to measure density of liquids and percent of solutions, such as the alcoholic content of liquids or the radiator of an automobile. The hydrometer consists of a closed glass tube, blown at one end and having a long stem at the other. The blown end is filled with a heavy weight (usually mercury or shot) to keep it erect when floated in a liquid. The long stem is internally calibrated with a graduated scale. For increased accuracy, there are hydrometers calibrated for use in light liquids and others for heavy liquids.

(1) *Theory of the hydrometer.* All floating bodies displace their own weight of a liquid in which they are immersed and sink to a depth proportionate to the volume of liquid displaced. Since this volume equals the weight of the immersed object, specific gravity can be determined by comparison of the volumes displaced. Thus a hydrometer is marked 1.000 at the level it sinks in distilled water at normal temperature. The scale is then carried above and below the 1.000 mark. When the instrument is placed in a different liquid, the specific gravity of that liquid can be read directly from the scale.

(2) *Testing the hydrometer.* Do not accept hydrometers as you receive them. Always test them first. By immersing your hydrometer in a number of liquids of known specific gravity, including water, you can observe its degree of accuracy. In the event a particular hydrometer shows consistent deviation of one or two points, you need not discard it as useless. Make a notation of the deviation on its box and merely add or subtract the error from the reading as you use it.

(3) *Hydrometer jar.* The hydrometer is generally floated in a hydrometer jar to take the reading (fig. 2-8). This device lessens the amount of liquid necessary for a reading because it is tall and narrow. It also facilitates cooling of the liquid to specified temperature, the jar being easily immersed in ice water.

(4) *Other applications of the hydrometer:*

(a) Urinometer—this hydrometer has a special scale for the determination of specific gravity of urine.

(b) Saccharometer—generally measures the percent of syrups rather than the specific gravity.

(c) Alcoholometer—determines alcoholic strength of hydroalcoholic solutions.

(d) Lovi's beads—also called specific gravity beads, are balloon-like, hollow globes of glass. They are of different sizes and weights and have a specific gravity number etched on their sides. When dropped into a liquid, those heavier than the liquid sink to the bottom; the ones lighter than the liquid float to the top; and the one which hovers in the liquid, neither floating nor sinking, represents the specific gravity. They must be used at a definite temperature for which they have been calibrated.

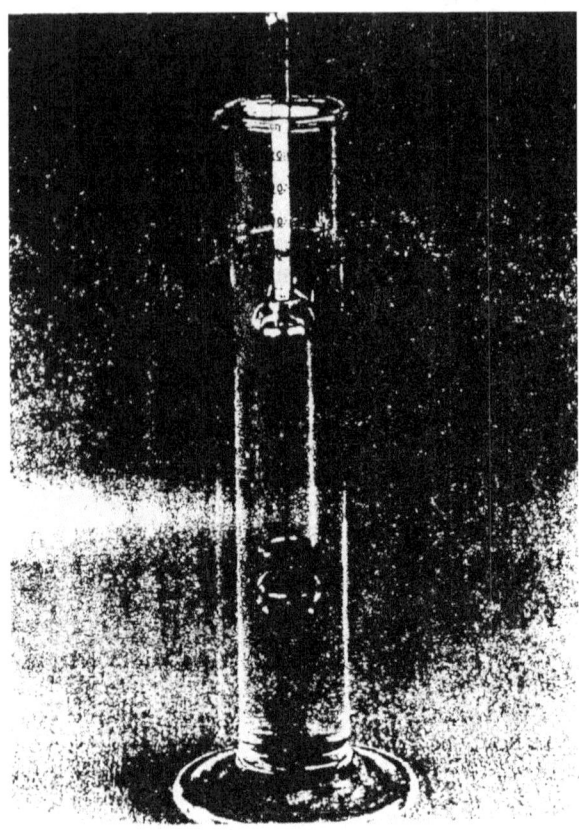

Figure 8. Hydrometer and jar.

37. Specific gravity of solids. Although various procedures must be used for determining the specific gravity of different solids, the formula used is always the same:

$$\text{Sp. Gr.} = \frac{\text{weight of solid in air}}{\text{weight of equal volume of water}}$$

Because of slight variations of technique necessary to establish the specific gravity of solids with different physical properties, we will break solids into groups according to their solubility and weight relative to water. Thus we have—
- Solids insoluble in and heavier than water.
- Solids soluble in and heavier than water.
- Solids insoluble in and lighter than water.
- Solids soluble in and lighter than water.

  a. Solids insoluble in and heavier than water.

  (1) When solid is a single piece. First, consider a solid in one piece, such as a block of metal or a strip of wire. The easiest method for determining specific gravity of a single piece of solid insoluble in and heavier than water is by using a balance.

- *Step 1.* Accurately weigh the sample to be tested on a good Rx or analytical balance and record this weight as the weight of the substance in air.

- *Step 2.* Attach a horsehair or fine, water-proofed, silk thread to the sample and to the beam of the scale. Immerse the sample in a beaker of water so that it is covered by the water, but not touching the bottom or sides of the beaker. The weight of the sample must be entirely supported by the beam of the balance. Make sure no air bubbles are attached to the sample which would provide buoyancy and make the weighing in water inaccurate. Record the weight of the sample in the water.

- *Step 3.* Apply the formula. *For example,* if a sample of copper weighs 10.52 Gm. in air and 9.34 Gm. when suspended in water, to find the specific gravity of the copper:

Weight in air   = 10.52 Gm.
Weight in water   9.34 Gm.
                 ─────────
                 1.18 = loss of weight in water

$$\text{Sp. Gr.} = \frac{\text{weight in air}}{\text{weight of equal volume of water}}$$

Since the loss of weight in water equals the weight of an equal volume of water, substitute in the formula:

$$\text{Sp. Gr.} = \frac{10.52}{1.18}$$

Sp. Gr. = 8.92 (copper)

  (2) When solid is fragmentary. Another method of determining the specific gravity of solids insoluble in and heavier than water is by the use of a pycnometer. This method is convenient when the solid is in fragments or smaller particles.

- *Step 1.* Weigh the sample in air and record the weight.

- *Step 2.* Drop the material into a tared pycnometer and fill with distilled water at 25° C. Weigh again, making sure that no water remains on the exterior of the vessel. This weight represents the weight of the pycnometer, the water, and the sample. Subtracting the tare weight, you have the weight of the sample plus the water in the bottle.

- *Step 3.* Apply the formula. *For example,* a sample weighing 10.5 Gm. is placed in a pyconometer which has been determined to hold

100 Gm. of water. You determine the weight of the sample plus the water plus the bottle to be 206.2 Gm. The tare weight of the bottle is 100 Gm.

```
  206.2 Gm. weight of bottle, water, sample
- 100.0 Gm. weight of bottle
  ─────────
  106.2 Gm. weight of water and sample
   10.5 Gm. weight of sample in air
  ─────────
  100.0 Gm. weight of water held by bottle
  110.5 Gm. weight of water plus sample
- 106.2 Gm. weight of water and immersed sample
  ─────────
    4.3 Gm. loss of weight in water
```

$$\text{Sp. Gr.} = \frac{10.5}{4.3} = 2.442, \text{ the specific gravity}$$

NOTE

The specific gravity of insoluble powders can also be determined by this method. Care should be taken to shake the powder with a quantity of water before filling the pycnometer to eliminate air bubbles and the error they can cause.

b. Solids insoluble in and lighter than water. The problem here is to make the solid sink into the water so that you can find out how much water it displaces. A weight or sinker, insoluble in water and heavy enough to cause the lighter sample to sink beneath the surface, can be attached. Since the loss of weight in water of the sample and sinker combined equals their total individual losses, it will be easy then to determine the loss of weight of the sample.

Example: A block of wax weighs 21.5 Gm. in the air. To this you attach a lead sinker which you have predetermined to lose 1.1 Gm. when immersed in water. Together they lose 25.8 grams when immersed in water. What is the specific gravity of the wax?

● *Step 1.*

Loss of weight of wax + sinker	=	25.8 Gm.
Loss of weight of sinker	−	1.1 Gm.
Loss of weight of wax	=	24.7 Gm.
Weight of wax in air	=	21.5 Gm.

● *Step 2.* Apply the formula.

$$\text{Sp. Gr.} \frac{21.5}{24.7}$$

$$\text{Sp. Gr.} = 0.87$$

c. Solids soluble in and heavier than water. The problem here is solubility. By substituting a liquid in which the sample is not soluble for the water, you can then determine by proportion what the loss of weight in water would be. The following proportion will apply:

$$\frac{\text{Sp. Gr. of oil}}{\text{Sp. Gr. of water}} :: \frac{\text{loss of weight in oil}}{\text{loss of weight in water}}$$

Example: 20.311 Gm. of Copper Sulfate immersed in an oil having a specific gravity of 0.865 filling a 100 Gm. pycnometer weighs 98.859 Gm. Find the specific gravity of copper sulfate.

● *Step 1.*

Weight of CuSO$_4$ in air	=	20.311 Gm.
Weight of oil in pycnom.	=	86.5 (100 × 0.865)
Weight of CuSO$_4$ + oil		106.811 Gm.

Weight of oil + immersed CuSO$_4$	=	98.859 Gm.
Weight of oil displaced		7.952 Gm.

● *Step 2.* Substitute in proportion.

$$\frac{\text{Sp. Gr. of oil}}{\text{Sp. Gr. of water}} :: \frac{\text{loss of weight in oil}}{\text{loss of weight in water}}$$

$$\frac{0.865}{1} :: \frac{7.952}{x}$$

$$865x = 7952$$

$$x = 9.193, \text{ the loss of weight in water}$$

● *Step 3.* Substitute in Sp. Gr. formula.

$$\text{Sp. Gr.} = \frac{20.311}{9.193}$$

$$\text{Sp. Gr.} = 2.209$$

NOTE

If the copper sulfate were in one solid lump, you could measure the loss of weight in oil directly by suspending it from a balance into the oil.

d. Solids soluble in and lighter than water. Here, the problem, and not a slight one, is to find a liquid lighter than the solid and one in which it is not soluble. When this is accomplished, the procedure is the same for solids soluble in and heavier than water (*c* above).

38. Application of specific gravity to pharmaceutical problems. Specific gravity, when known, is of great assistance to us as pharmacists in reducing metric and apothecary volumes to weight and, conversely, in reducing weights to volumes.

a. Metric.
- 1 ml. of water weighs 1 Gm.
- Sp. Gr. of water is 1.000.
- 1 ml. of any liquid with Sp. Gr. of 1.000 weighs 1 Gm.
- 1 ml. of a liquid with Sp. Gr. of 2.000 weighs (1 x 2.000) 2 Gm.
- 1 ml. of a liquid with Sp. Gr. of 1.5 weighs 1 x 1.5 or 1.5 Gm.

Therefore, the volume in ml. times specific gravity = weight in Gm.

   (1) Example: What is the weight in grams of 1 liter of glycerin (Sp. Gr. 1.25)?

- *Step 1.* 1 liter = 1000 ml.

- *Step 2.* 1000 ml. x 1.25 = 1250 Gm., the weight of 1 liter of glycerin.

   (2) Example: How many ml. of chloroform are there in 1480 Gm.? (Sp. Gr. of chloroform = 1.48).

   x ml. x 1.48 = 1480 Gm.

$$x = \frac{1480}{1.48} = 1000 \text{ ml. or 1 liter of chloroform}$$

b. Apothecary. There is no convenient weight-to-volume comparison in the apothecary system. However, you may derive a working formula from the steps below.

- *Step 1.* In the metric system, 1 gram of water or any liquid with a specific gravity of 1.000, has a corresponding volume of 1 ml. In the apothecary system, a fluidounce of water or any fluid with a specific gravity of 1.000 does not weigh 1 ounce, nor does a fluidrachm weigh a drachm, nor a minim weigh a grain.

- *Step 2.* BUT, 1 fluidounce of water at 25° C. weighs 454.6 grains. Since there are 480 minims in 1 fluidounce, a minim of water weighs 454.6 ÷ 480 = 0.95 grain.

- *Step 3.* 1 fluidounce of any liquid having a specific gravity of 1.000 weighs 454.6 grain. 1 fluidounce of any liquid having a specific gravity of 2.000 weighs 454.6 x 2.

- *Step 4.* Conclusion. 1 fluidounce of any liquid weighs (in grains) 454.6 x specific gravity. Thus the following formula:
454.6 x Sp. Gr. x number of fluidounces = weight in grains.

   (1) Example: How much does f℥ii, ℨiv of glycerin weigh? Sp. Gr. of glycerin is 1.25.

- *Step 1.* f℥ii, ℨiv = 2.5 fluidounces.

- *Step 2.* Substitute in formula:
454.6 x 1.25 x 2.5 = weight in grains

```
   454.6          568.25
 x  1.25        x   2.5
  22730          284125
   9092          113650
   4546          1420.625, weight of glycerin
 568.250
```

- *Step 3.* Convert to highest terms.
1420.625 rounded off (.625 → .63 grains)
20 gr./Ә, so 1420 ÷ 20 = 71 Ә
3 Ә/ℨ , so 71 ÷ 3 = 23 ℨ + 2 Ә remainder
8 ℨ/℥ , so 23 ÷ 8 = 2 ℥ + 7 ℨ remainder

- *Step 4.* Collect the amounts.
℥ii ℨvii Әii gr ss(.63)

   (2) Example: What is the volume of 250 grains of a liquid with a specific gravity of 0.942?

- *Step 1.* Formula.
454.6 x 0.942 x y (No. fluidounces) = weight in grains
454.6 x 0.942 x y = 250

```
      0.942
    x 454.6
      5652
      3768
      4710
      3768
    428.2332
```

y(428.233) = 250

$$y = \frac{250}{428.233}$$

y = .583 fluidounce

- *Step 2.* Reduce to correct terms.
8 fℨ = 1 f℥
therefore, .583 x 8 = 4.664 fluidrachms
60 minims = 1 fℨ
therefore, .664 x 60 = 40 minims

- *Step 3.* Combine the quantities:
fℨ iv ♏ x l

39. Specific volume

a. Identification. Specific volume is much like specific gravity, except the comparison is between volumes rather than weights. Specific volume can be described as the ratio of the volume of one substance to the volume of an equal weight of a standard substance. As in specific gravity, the standard is water and the standard temperature is 25° C.

Since Sp. Gr. = $\dfrac{\text{weight of substance in air}}{\text{weight of equal volume of water}}$

Sp. Vol. = $\dfrac{\text{volume of substance}}{\text{volume of equal weight of water}}$

Then, Specific Gravity = $\dfrac{1}{\text{Sp. Vol.}}$ and

Sp. Vol. = $\dfrac{1}{\text{Sp. Gr.}}$; they are reciprocals

b. Sample problems.
(1) Problem: What is the specific volume of 750 Gm. of chloroform measuring 510.2 ml.?

- *Step 1.* Volume of chloroform = 510.2 ml.
  Volume of equal weight water = 750.0 ml.

- *Step 2.* Substitute in formula

  Sp. Vol. = $\dfrac{\text{volume of substance}}{\text{volume of equal weight water}}$

  Sp. Vol. = $\dfrac{510.2}{750}$

  Sp. Vol = 0.68

(2) Problem: Using the information in the previous problem, what is the specific gravity of chloroform?
Using the reciprocal formula:

Sp. Gr. = $\dfrac{1}{\text{Sp. Vol.}}$

Sp. Gr. = $\dfrac{1}{0.68}$

Sp. Gr. = 1.47, answer

```
       1.47
68/100.00
   68
   32 0
   27 2
    4 80
    4 76
```

40. Density

a. Identification. Density is the ratio between weight and volume of a substance; or, density = weight divided by volume, and is expressed not as a relative number, as specific gravity was, but with specific units as Gm./ml., lb/cu.ft., or gr./fl.oz.

From the formula:

$D = \dfrac{w}{v}$, we see that if we know density and volume we can determine weight; knowing density and weight, we can find volume; and knowing weight and volume, we can find density.

b. Sample problems.
(1) Problem: What is the density of alcohol if 250 ml. weigh 200 Gm.?

Density = $\dfrac{\text{weight}}{\text{volume}}$

$D = \dfrac{200}{250}$

$D = 0.80$ Gm./ml.

(2) Problem: How many ml. of mercury (density 13.6) would there be in a sample weighing 2000 Gm.?

$D = \dfrac{w}{v}$

$13.6 = \dfrac{2000}{v}$

$13.6\,v = 2000$

$v = \dfrac{2000}{13.6}$

$v = 147.06$ ml.

41. Temperature

a. Definition. What exactly is temperature? Temperature can be stated as being the degree of hotness or lack of hotness, or the *intensity of heat*. Relative temperatures can be sensed by touch in some cases, but the sense of touch can be very misleading. A piece of cloth and a piece of metal, although exactly the same temperature will feel differently to the touch. The cloth will not seem as warm or as cold as the metal. This is due to the rate at which the substance dissipates heat.

b. Measurement of temperature. Temperature, therefore, must be measured by a device which gives accurate degrees of heat. Such instruments are called thermometers. The thermometer is based on the principle of expansion and contraction of substances with change in temperature. The most common thermometers utilize alcohol or mercury. In order for readings obtained from expansion and contraction to be valid, the expansion and contraction must be uniform.

c. Liquid thermometer. The liquid thermometer consists of a fine capillary tube, hermetically sealed, with a bulb at one end. The tube is filled to a point on the capillary, the bulb serving as a reservoir. Upon elevating the temperature, the liquid expands and rises in the tube to a new level. Thus, calibrating the tube with known constant temperatures and dividing the space between with equal degrees, we have an instrument that will measure temperature. Figure 2-9 shows two liquid thermometers discussed below.

42. Temperature calculation. There are two different scales by which liquid thermometers can be calibrated—the Centigrade scale and the Fahrenheit scale.

a. Centigrade. The Centigrade thermometer is so calibrated that the melting point of ice is 0° C. and the boiling point of water is 100° C. By this scale, there is a difference of 100 degrees between the freezing and boiling points of water. The Centigrade scale has been adopted by the USP and NF as the official temperature standard. In fact, it is the standard temperature measuring device the world over.

b. Fahrenheit. The Fahrenheit thermometer is calibrated so that 32° F. is the melting point of ice and 212° F. is the boiling point of water. The difference between freezing and boiling on this scale is 180°. The Fahrenheit scale is used mainly for household purposes.

c. Importance of stating the scale. Because of the great difference between these two scales, you can see the importance of always stating which scale you are using when referring to a temperature. By itself, 40° means nothing; 40° Fahrenheit is approximately 4.4° Centigrade; 40° Centigrade is 104° Fahrenheit, a considerable difference.

d. Absolute temperature. We, as pharmacists, will not deal with the absolute temperature scale; however, you should be familiar with what it is. Remember only that *absolute* degree equals Centigrade degrees plus 273°. Expressed as a formula this becomes—

$$A° = C° + 273°.$$

43. Temperature conversion. Knowing that the range in degrees between the freezing and boiling points of water is 100° in the Centigrade scale and 180° in the Fahrenheit scale, it is obvious that one Centigrade degree is equal to 1.8 (9/5), the size of a Fahrenheit degree. Therefore, a 5-degree change in Centigrade temperature is a 9-degree change in the Fahrenheit scale. Since 0° C. equals 32° F., 1° C. must equal 32° plus 9/5° or 1.8°, or 33.8° F. Thus, we can derive several formulas. However, the basic formula is: 9C = 5F − 160, or 5F = 9C + 160.

a. Example: Convert −5° Centigrade to Fahrenheit.

- *Step 1.* Formula: 5F = 9C + 160

- *Step 2.* Substitute: 5F = 9 (−5) + 160
    5F = −45 + 160
    5F = 115
    F = 115 ÷ 5
    F = 23° F

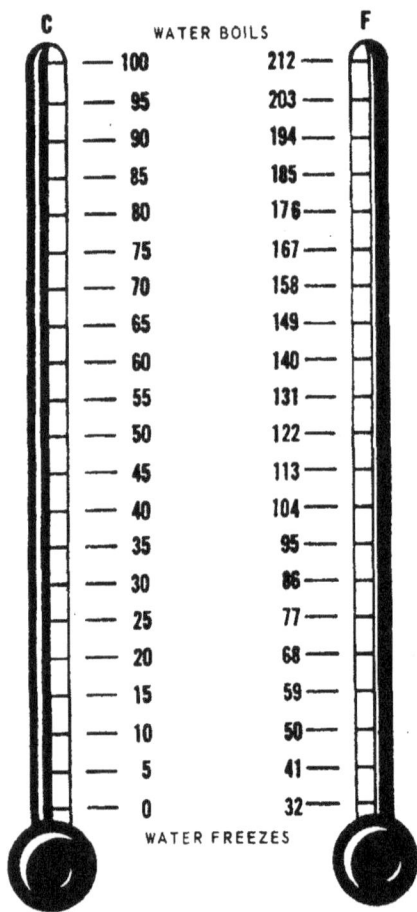

Figure 9. Thermometer comparison.

b. Example: Convert −40° Fahrenheit to Centigrade.

- *Step 1.* Formula: 9C = 5F − 160
- *Step 2.* Substitute: 9C = 5 (−40) − 160
  9C = −200 − 160
  9C = −360
  C = −360 ÷ 9
  C = −40° C

   c. Example: Convert 80° Fahrenheit to Centigrade.

- *Step 1.* Formula: 9C = 5F − 160
- *Step 2.* Substitute: 9C = 5(80) − 160
  9C = 400 − 160
  9C = 240
  C = 240 ÷ 9
  C = 26.6° C

44. Dosage

   a. Importance of dosage calculation to the pharmacist. When a prescription reaches the pharmacist from the desk of a prescriber, the ingredients are specified, the quantities listed (perhaps in specific amounts, perhaps as ratio, perhaps as percentages), and the instructions to the patient are written in Latin, in pharmaceutical or medical terminology. The pharmacist must (1) fill the prescription, (2) check the prescriber for possible error of amounts and dosage, and (3) write the directions upon the label in terms which can be easily understood by the patient. For these reasons, an accurate knowledge of dosage is mandatory for the pharmacist. Imagine the consequences of the following:

   (1) Error in converting a percent ingredient to the specific amount.

   (2) Prescriber's inadvertent error in amount of ingredient to be used in preparation of a medicinal (with the accompanying error of the pharmacist not observing the error).

   (3) Prescriber's error in calculation of dosage (again combined with the pharmacist's missing the error). Although errors are the exception rather than the rule, the pharmacist must be forever on his guard against them. It is not his privilege to look for errors, but his *duty*. The pharmacist is held responsible equally with the erring physician. Overdose, even though it may originate at the prescriber, if not corrected by the pharmacy technician may constitute negligence.

   b. Approximate household equivalents. The approximate household equivalents shown in table 2-8 are useful in making calculations for number of doses in a medication and for translating directions into terms understandable to the patient. These approximate equivalents are in obvious discrepancy due to approximating equivalency between three different measures. In table 2-8, one teasp., 1 f ʒ (approx 4 ml.) and 5 ml. are not equal at all. However, the directions to the patient cannot read "Take 1 drachm" or "4 ml." or "5 ml." They must be written in some language that all literate persons can understand—thus, "one teaspoonful."

   c. Medicine glass. Because of inaccuracy in household equivalents and because household spoons, cups, and glasses vary considerably in size, the patient should be strongly advised to purchase a medicine glass (fig. 2-10) for accurate dosage.

   d. Calculation of dosage. Some of the dosage calculations you will be making most frequently are listed below. The following proportion can be established which will aid in solving dosage problems:

$$\text{Total doses} = \frac{\text{total amount}}{\text{size of each dose}}$$

   (1) Calculating the size of an individual dose. When given the total amount of medication and the number of doses to be made, the size of each can be calculated by dividing. *Example:* A

Table 8. Approximate Household Equivalents

Metric measure	Apothecary equivalent (approximate)	Household measure
2 ml	f ʒ ss	½ teaspoonful
5 ml	f ʒ i	1 teaspoonful
8 ml	f ʒ ii	1 dessertspoonful
15 ml	f ʒ iv	1 tablespoonful
30 ml	f ʒ viii (f ℥ i)	2 tablespoonfuls
60 m	f ℥ ii	1 wineglassful
120 ml	f ℥ iv	1 teacupful
240 ml	f ℥ viii	1 tumblerful

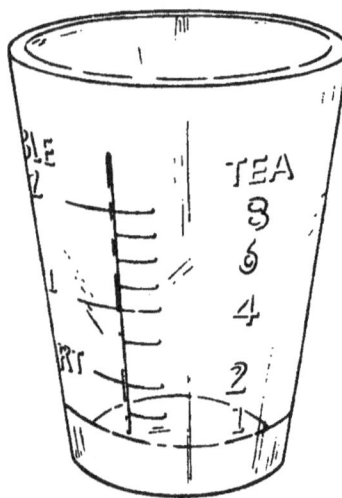

Figure 10. A medicine glass.

particular medication is to be taken 4 times daily for 1 week, and a total of 280 grains is being dispensed. What is the amount of this medication in a single dose?

- *Step 1.* What is the total number of doses?
  4 doses daily x 7 days = 28 doses, total

- *Step 2.* Formula.
  $$\text{Total doses} = \frac{\text{total amount}}{\text{size of each dose}}$$

- *Step 3.* Substitute—
  $$28 = \frac{280 \text{ gr.}}{x}$$
  $$28x = 280$$
  $$x = 10 \text{ grains in each dose.}$$

NOTE

The answer will always be in the same denomination as the total amount, or if the total amount is the unknown, in the same denomination as the individual dose.

(2) *Calculating number of doses.* The number of doses in a specific amount can be calculated if you are given the total amount and the size of the dose.

(a) *Example:* How many doses of 5 grains each will result from a total of 75 grains of total medication?

- *Step 1.* Formula.
  $$\text{Total doses} = \frac{\text{total amount}}{\text{size of each dose}}$$

- *Step 2.* Substitute.
  $$x = \frac{75 \text{ gr.}}{5}$$
  $$x = 15 \text{ doses}$$

(b) *Example:* If the dose of a medication is to be one-half fluidrachm, how many doses will a patient receive, given an 8-ounce bottle of medication?

- *Step 1.* Since there are 8 fluidrachms to the fluidounce, 8 fluidounces would contain 8 x 8 = 64 fluidrachms.

- *Step 2.* Formula.
  $$\text{Total doses} = \frac{\text{total amount}}{\text{size of each dose}}$$

- *Step 3.* Substitute.
  $$x = \frac{64 \text{ fluidrachms}}{.5}$$
  $$x = 128 \text{ doses, answer}$$

(3) *Calculating total amount of medication.* If you know the size of the dose and the number of doses prescribed, you can determine the total medication to be dispensed.

Example: A patient is to receive 1 fluidounce of whisky morning, noon, and night for an indefinite period of time. What quantity would be dispensed for 1 week's medication?

- *Step 1.* 1 ounce dose x 3 doses per day x 7 days per week equals 21 ounces. The formula may also be used as shown in step 2 below.

- *Step 2.* Formula.
  $$\text{Total doses} = \frac{\text{total amount}}{\text{size of each dose}}$$
  $$21 = \frac{x}{1}$$
  $$x = 21 \text{ ounces, answer}$$

(4) *Calculating amount of a single ingredient.* The amount of a single ingredient present in a dose of a mixture of several medicinal agents can be determined by dividing the amount of that ingredient by the total doses.

(a) *Example:* Calculate the amount of *each* ingredient in a single dose of the following prescription.

    Rx Acetylsalicylic acid   ℨii Ɔi gr vii
       Acetophenetidin   ℨi   Ɔii gr v
       Caffeine   gr xss
       M. Ft. M.
       Div in caps, no. xxi
       Sig: Cap i q 4 h, prn.

- *Step 1.* Reduce all ingredients to *grains*.
  Acetylsalicylic acid equals
    2 x 60 grains (per drachm)   = 120 gr.
    1 x 20 grains (per scruple) = 20 gr.
    7 grains   =   7 gr.
                                   147 gr.
  Acetophenetidin equals
    1 x 60 grains (per drachm)   = 60 gr.
    2 x 20 grains (per scruple) = 40 gr.
    5 grains   =   5 gr.
                                   105 gr.
  Caffeine equals
    10 1/2 grains   = 10.5 gr.

- *Step 2.* You know that the total amount is for 21 capsules; therefore, the amount in a single capsule would be—

$$\text{Total doses} = \frac{\text{total amount}}{\text{size of each dose}}$$

$21 = \frac{147}{x}$ = 7 grains acetylsalicylic acid per capsule

$21 = \frac{105}{x}$ = 5 grains acetophenetidin per capsule

$21 = \frac{10.5}{x}$ = 1/2 grain caffeine per capsule

NOTE

To check this prescription for possible errors, consult the USP or Remington for the dose of each of the ingredients and compare the dose with the amounts you have calculated to be in each capsule.

(b) *Example:* A solution contains 4/5 grain of a potent drug in 4 ounces. What dose must be given to provide 1/120 grain of the drug?

- *Step 1.* Formula.

$$\text{Total doses} = \frac{\text{total amount}}{\text{size of each dose}}$$

- *Step 2* Substitute.

$$x \text{ doses} = \frac{\frac{4}{15}}{\frac{1}{120}}$$

- *Step 3.* Remember that you can divide fractions by inverting the divisor and multiplying. Thus,

$$x \text{ doses} = \frac{4}{15} \times \frac{120}{1}$$

$$x = \frac{480}{15} = 32 \text{ doses}$$

- *Step 4.* Since you are to get 32 doses from 4 ounces, each dose must be one fluidrachm (8 fluidrachms = 1 ounce).

e. *Children's doses.* Enough emphasis cannot be placed upon the calculation of dosage for children. Because of their size, weight, and incomplete development, they are not able to tolerate as much medication as adults. Although many factors besides weight and age play an important part in dosage, only these two will be discussed here. (Chapter 9 explains dosage factors in more detail.)

(1) *Formulas for calculating children's doses.* Several formulas can be employed for calculating doses for children and infants; however, because of different degrees of response by children to different medications (e.g., children are extremely susceptible to morphine), it is best to become familiar with the correct doses through experience and to memorize doses as they present themselves. If at all in doubt about the size of a dose, ALWAYS check with the pharmacy officer or the prescriber. The most generally used formulas for calculation of doses for children are—

(a) *Young's rule* (most widely used).

$$\frac{\text{child's age}}{\text{child's age} + 12} \times \text{adult dose} = \text{child's dose}$$

(b) *Clark's rule.*

$$\frac{\text{weight of child (lb)}}{150} \times \text{adult dose} = \text{child's dose}$$

(2) *Example problems.* Study the following examples carefully to see the application of the above rules.

(a) *Example:* What would be the dose of elixir of phenobarbital for a child 3 years old? (Elixir phenobarbital contains 400 mg. of phenobarbital per 100 ml. Adult dose of phenobarbital is 30 mg., up to 4 times a day.) Use Young's rule.

- *Step 1.* Rule.

$$\frac{\text{child's age}}{\text{child's age} + 12} \times \text{adult dose} = \text{child's dose}$$

- *Step 2.* Substitute.

$$\frac{3}{3+12} \times 30 \text{ mg.} = \text{child's dose}$$

$$\frac{90}{15} = 6 \text{ mg., the child's dose}$$

- *Step 3.* Since 100 ml. of phenobarbital elixir contains 400 mg., 1 ml. would contain 4 mg. Therefore; 1:x :: 4:6.

$$4x = 6$$
$$x = 1.5 \text{ ml., the dose for 3-year-old child.}$$

(b) Example: What would be the dose of tetracycline hydrochloride for a 3-year-old girl weighing 30 pounds? Usual adult dose is 500 mg. Use Clark's rule.

- *Step 1.* Formula.

$$\frac{\text{weight of child (lb)}}{150} \times \text{adult dose} = \text{child's dose}$$

- *Step 2.* Substitute.

$$\frac{30}{150} \times 500 \text{ mg.} = \text{child's dose}$$

$$\frac{15,000}{150} = 100 \text{ mg., the child's dose}$$

45. Concentration and dilution. Many times in pharmacy it is necessary to dilute or concentrate a substance in order to dispense the right dosage; the dilution of nose drops is one of the most frequently seen examples. Phenylephrine hydrochloride solution is a standard nose drop preparation. Its strength as it comes to us is 1 percent. Most of the prescriptions for phenylephrine solution will call for 1/4 percent. You can see, then, that it will have to be diluted before dispensing.

a. Mechanics of dilution. If 1 ounce of a 1 percent-solution of phenylephrine hydrochloride solution was diluted to a new volume of 2 ounces, the percent of the new solution would be 1/2 of the original 1 percent, that is, 1/2 percent. Perhaps it will be more apparent if you consider that 1 ounce of a 1-percent solution contains approximately 4.5 grains of active ingredient. By diluting the solution to a volume of 2 ounces, you still have only 4.5 grains of active ingredient in a volume of 2 ounces. Thus, you have halved the percentage. If the active ingredient remains constant and the volume of the solution increases, the percentage decreases. And if the active ingredient remains constant and the volume of the solution decreases, the percentage increases. The percentage strength and the volume of a solution are inversely proportional to each other.

b. Concentration–dilution proportion. Since volume and percentage strength of solutions are inversely proportional, the following formula or proportion applies.

$$\frac{\text{\% concentration of original solution}}{\text{\% concentration of new solution}} :: \frac{\text{new volume}}{\text{original volume}}$$

This proportion can be used to solve any concentration or dilution problem arising in the pharmacy.

(1) Example: You have 30 ml. of a 10-percent solution and want to make a 1-percent solution. To what volume must you dilute the original solution? Substituting in the proportion you have—

$$\frac{10 \text{ (original \%)}}{1 \text{ (new \%)}} :: \frac{x \text{ (unknown new volume)}}{30 \text{ (original new volume)}}$$

$$x = 300 \text{ ml., the new volume}$$

In a practical situation, then, you would dilute the original 30 ml. of 10-percent solution to a total volume of 300 ml. to prepare the desired 1-percent solution.

(2) Example: Make a 4-percent solution from 60 ml. of a 2-percent solution by concentrating the volume. Again, substituting in the proportion, you have—

$$\frac{2\%}{4\%} :: \frac{x}{60}$$
$$4x = 120$$
$$x = 30 \text{ ml.}$$

You must concentrate the 60 ml. of 2-percent solution to a new volume of 30 ml. in order to obtain the 4-percent solution.

46. Alligation. Alligation is a process for finding the value of a combination containing known quantities of known strengths; *for example,* to determine the strength of a solution resulting from the mixture of 100 ml. of 20-percent alcohol and

20 ml. of 10-percent alcohol. Actually, alligation is two different processes, alligation medial and alligation alternate. Alligation medial is used for determining percentage strength and alligation alternate for proportional number of parts.

  a. Alligation medial. Alligation medial is used in determining the percentage strength of a mixture of two or more ingredients of different strengths. Alligation medial can also be used to determine the resulting specific gravity of a mixture of two or more substances with different specific gravities.

  (1) Example: What percentage of codeine sulfate is contained in a mixture of 60 grams of a 15-percent codeine powder and 15 grams of a 40-percent codeine powder?

- *Step 1.* Find the amount of codeine sulfate in the total mixture.

  60 x .15 = 9.0 Gm. of codeine sulfate
  15 x .40 = 6.0 Gm. of codeine sulfate
  15.0 Gm. total codeine in mixture

- *Step 2.* Find the weight of the total mixture.

  60 Gm. + 15 Gm. = 75 Gm. total weight of mixture

- *Step 3.* Divide the amount of codeine by the total weight to find the percent of codeine in the mixture.

  $\frac{15.0}{75.0}$ = .20 or 20% codeine sulfate

  (2) Example: You prepare a mixture of 3 ounces of liquid A and 13 ounces of liquid B. What is the cost per ounce of the resulting mixture if liquid A costs $4.00 per pint and liquid B costs $1.44 per pint?

- *Step 1.* Find the cost per ounce of each ingredient.

  A = $4.00/pint ÷ 16 = $ .25/ounce
  B = $1.44/pint ÷ 16 = $ .09/ounce

- *Step 2.* Find the number of ounces in the total mixture.

  3 ounces of A + 13 ounces of B = 16 ounces

- *Step 3.* Find the total cost of these two ingredients.

  3 ounces at $0.25 = $ .75
  13 ounces at $0.09 = $1.17
  $1.92 total cost of mixture

- *Step 4.* Find the cost per ounce of the mixture.

  $1.92 ÷ 16 = $0.12, cost per ounce

  (3) Example: What is the specific gravity of a mixture of 250 ml. of Glycerin (Sp. Gr. 1.25) and 500 ml. of chloroform (Sp. Gr. 1.48)?

- *Step 1.* Find the number of grams in each of the volumes.

  250 ml. x 1.25 = 312.5 Gm. of glycerin
  500 ml. x 1.48 = 740.00 Gm. of chloroform

- *Step 2.* Find the total volume and total weight of the mixture.

  250 ml. + 500 ml. = 750 ml., total volume
  312.5 Gm. + 740 Gm. = 1052.5 Gm., total weight

- *Step 3.* Divide weight by volume to find Sp. Gr.

  $\frac{1052.5}{750}$ = 1.403, the Sp. Gr. of mixture

  b. Alligation alternate. Alligation alternate is a method of determining the proportionate number of parts of two or more ingredients of known strength when they are to be mixed to form a desired strength. The parts can then be changed to represent volume or weight. A substance of greater strength is mixed with one of lesser strength to form a mixture of a strength somewhere between that of the two ingredients. For example, 50-percent alcohol can be mixed with 25-percent alcohol to produce 30-percent alcohol. It is not possible to mix 50-percent alcohol with 25-percent alcohol to get less than 25-percent or more than 50-percent alcohol. The increase in percentage from the smaller ingredient to the percentage desired, equals the parts of the higher percent ingredient, and the decrease in percentage of the higher to the desired equals the parts of the lower percent ingredient.

  (1) Example: What must be the proportion of 50-percent alcohol and 25-percent alcohol, mixed to obtain 30-percent alcohol?

- *Step 1.* Examine the situation. We desire a 30-percent alcohol solution from a 50-percent and a 25-percent solution. The 50-percent solution is 20 percent too strong and the 25-percent solution is 5 percent too weak. In other words, the 50-percent solution must decrease 20 percent and the 25-percent increase 5 percent.

● *Step 2.* Prepare a diagram and place the percentage you desire at completion in the center block. Place the highest percent ingredient (50 percent) on the left and the lowest percent ingredient (25 percent) on the right.

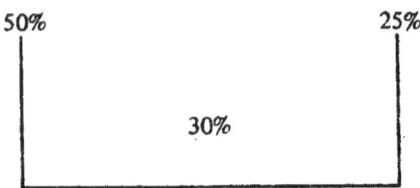

● *Step 3.* Subtract the percent you desire (center block) from the high percent and place your answer below the low percent. This answer represents the parts of the LOW percent you will need to make the desired strength solution.

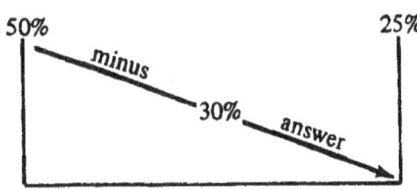

● *Step 4.* Subtract the low percent from the desired percent (center block) and place your answer below the high percent. This answer represents the parts of the HIGH percent you will need to make the desired strength solution.

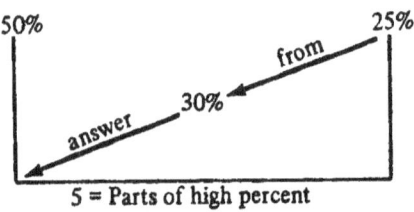

The paperwork from your completed problem, then, should look like this. It indicates that to make a 30-percent solution from 50-percent and 25-percent alcohol, you will need 5 parts of the 50 percent and 20 parts of the 25 percent.

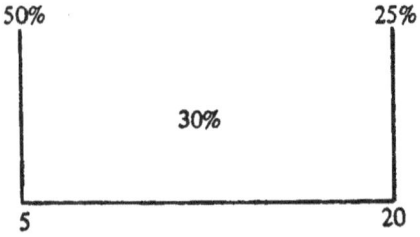

● *Step 5.* Express the number of parts in the denomination most suitable, such as ml., grains, grams, or ounces. Thus, 20 ml. of the 25 percent + 5 ml. of the 50 percent will make a 30-percent mixture; 20 ounces of the 25 percent + 5 ounces of the 50 percent will also make a 30-percent mixture.

  (2) Example: In what proportion must you mix 95-percent, 10-percent, 50-percent, and 30-percent alcohol to make 40-percent alcohol?

● *Step 1.* Examine the situation. You desire a 40-percent solution by combining so many parts each of 95 percent, 50 percent, 30 percent, and 10 percent.

● *Step 2.* Although the setup looks a little different because there are 4 ingredients in this problem, use the same procedure, that is, to subtract the lesser percents from the desired to get the number of parts, and to subtract the desired percent from the higher percents to get the number of parts. This problem has been broken down into four diagrams to show each segment of subtraction. However, the problem should be worked from one diagram.

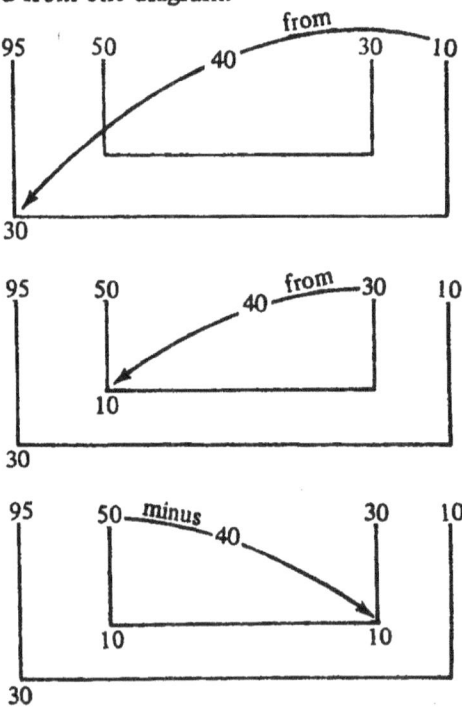

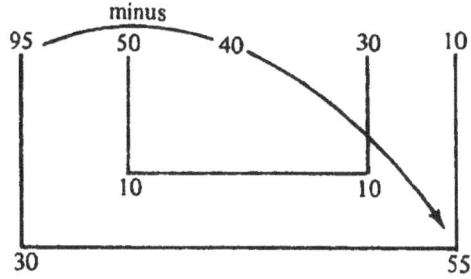

You therefore need—

> 30 parts of 95% alcohol
> 55 parts of 10% alcohol
> 10 parts of 50% alcohol
> 10 parts of 30% alcohol
> ---
> 105 parts of 40% alcohol

● *Step 3.* By expressing the parts as ounces, you mix 30 ounces of 95 percent, 55 ounces of 10 percent, 10 ounces of 50 percent, and 10 ounces of 30 percent to produce 105 ounces of 40-percent alcohol.

   (3) Example: How many ml. of 10-percent, 20-percent, and 30-percent sodium hydroxide solution must be mixed to make a quart of 25-percent solution?

● *Step 1.* Examine the situation. You desire a 25-percent solution from the combination of 10-percent, 20-percent, and 30-percent solutions of sodium hydroxide.

● *Step 2.* Set up.

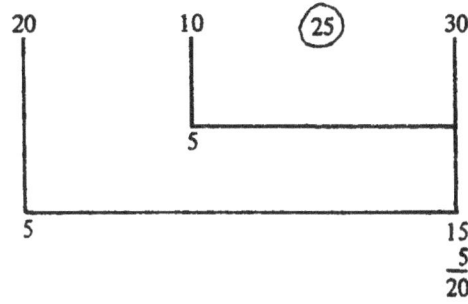

● *Step 3.* Thus you need—

> 5 parts of 20%
> 5 parts of 10%
> 20 parts of 30%
> ---
> 30 parts of 25% will result

● *Step 4.* Find what one part would equal. You know that there are 473 ml. in 1 pint, and therefore 946 ml. in 1 quart. The total number of ml. to be made is 946. You have a total of 30 parts of the solutions which are to equal 946 ml.; 1 part, then, would equal 946 ÷ 30 = 31.53 ml. per part.

● *Step 5.* Multiply the numbers of parts by the 31.53 ml. to find the number of ml. of each to be used.

$$31.53 \times 5 = 157.65 \text{ ml. of } 20\%$$
$$31.53 \times 5 = 157.65 \text{ ml. of } 10\%$$
$$31.53 \times 20 = 630.60 \text{ ml. of } 30\%$$

   (4) Example: How much water must be added to a pint of 95-percent ethyl alcohol to make 70-percent alcohol?

● *Step 1.* Examine the situation. You desire to make a 70-percent solution of alcohol from a 95-percent solution and a 0-percent solution (water).

● *Step 2.* Set up.

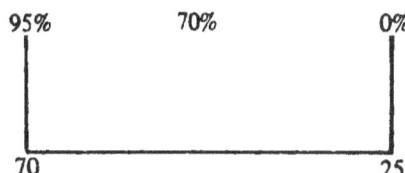

● *Step 3.* Thus you need—

> 70 parts of 95% alcohol
> 25 parts of 0% alcohol (water)
> ---
> 95 parts of 70% alcohol

● *Step 4.* Solve. One pint contains 473 ml.

$$70 : 473 :: 25 : x$$
$$70x = 473 \times 25$$
$$70x = 11{,}825$$
$$x = 168.93 \text{ ml. of water required.}$$

   (5) Example: How many ml. of a 60-percent sulfuric acid by volume solution must be added to 344 ml. of 30-percent sulfuric acid and 172 ml. of 15-percent sulfuric acid to make 50-percent sulfuric acid?

● *Step 1.* Examine the situation. You desire to make a 50-percent solution of sulfuric acid by combining 344 ml. of 30-percent sulfuric acid, 172 ml. of 15-percent sulfuric acid, and x number of ml. of 60-percent sulfuric acid.

● *Step 2.* Find the percent strength of the mixture formed by combining the acids of known strength and volume.

$$344 \times 0.30 = 103.2 \text{ Gm.}$$
$$\underline{172 \times 0.15} = \underline{25.8 \text{ Gm.}}$$
$$516 \text{ ml.} \qquad 129.0 \text{ Gm.}$$

$129.0 \div 516 = .25$, or 25%, the strength of the mixture of the two acids.

● *Step 3.* Set up for a mixture of the 25 percent and the 60 percent to be added.

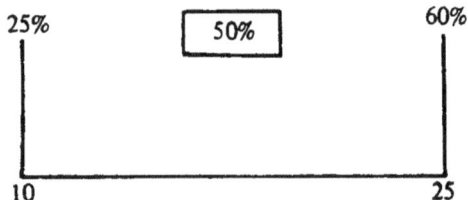

● *Step 4.* Thus you need—

25 parts of 60% sulfuric acid
10 parts of 25% sulfuric acid
―
35 parts of 50% sulfuric acid

● *Step 5.* Since you have 516 ml. of the 25-percent strength solution, which represents 10 parts, find how many ml. will represent 25 parts.

$$10 : 25 :: 516 : x$$
$$10x = 516 \times 25$$
$$10x = 12,900$$
$$x = 1,290 \text{ ml. of the 60% sulfuric acid required.}$$

www.ingramcontent.com/pod-product-compliance
Lightning Source LLC
Chambersburg PA
CBHW081822300426
44116CB00014B/2449